SPLINTING
AND CASTING

HANDBOOK OF SPLINTING AND CASTING

Stephen R. Thompson, MD, MEd, FRCSC
Fellow
Fowler Kennedy Sport Medicine Clinic
University of Western Ontario
London, Ontario, Canada

Dan A. Zlotolow, MD
Clinical Assistant Professor of Orthopaedics
Temple University School of Medicine
Shriners Hospital for Children of Philadelphia
Philadelphia, Pennsylvania

Photography by Brian O'Doherty

ELSEVIER
MOSBY

1600 John F. Kennedy Blvd.
Ste 1800
Philadelphia, PA 19103-2899

HANDBOOK OF SPLINTING AND CASTING   ISBN: 978-0-323-07802-3

Notices

Knowledge and best practice in this field are constantly changing. As new research and
experience broaden our understanding, changes in research methods, professional
practices, or medical treatment may become necessary. Practitioners and researchers must
always rely on their own experience and knowledge in evaluating and using any information,
methods, compounds, or experiments described herein. In using such information or
methods they should be mindful of their own safety and the safety of others, including
parties for whom they have a professional responsibility.

With respect to any drug or pharmaceutical products identified, readers are advised
to check the most current information provided (i) on procedures featured or (ii) by the
manufacturer of each product to be administered, to verify the recommended dose
or formula, the method and duration of administration, and contraindications. It is the
responsibility of practitioners, relying on their own experience and knowledge of their
patients, to make diagnoses, to determine dosages and the best treatment for each
individual patient, and to take all appropriate safety precautions.

To the fullest extent of the law, neither the Publisher nor the authors, contributors, or
editors, assume any liability for any injury and/or damage to persons or property as
a matter of products liability, negligence or otherwise, or from any use or operation of any
methods, products, instructions, or ideas contained in the material herein.

Library of Congress Cataloging-in-Publication Data

ISBN: 978-0-323-07802-3

Acquisitions Editor: James Merritt
Developmental Editor: Andrea Vosburgh
Publishing Services Manager: Patricia Tannian
Project Manager: Carrie Stetz
Design Direction: Ellen Zanolle

Printed in the United States of America
Last digit is the print number: 9 8 7 6 5 4 3 2 1

DEDICATION

For Shannon—Words cannot express my thankfulness for all that you have sacrificed to allow me to do this. With all my love.

Stephen R. Thompson

To Marie, the "world's most casted human being," who endured cast saw burns and hours of traction to make this project possible. My unending gratitude.

Dan A. Zlotolow

Preface

In many ways, it is unfortunate that a book detailing how to reduce, cast, and splint has not previously been published. We learned the techniques detailed in this book from a generation of orthopedists who relied almost entirely on their hands for diagnosing, reducing, and immobilizing fractures and dislocations. In the days before arthroscopy and MRI, specialized reduction maneuvers, splints, and casts were passed from teacher to pupil. Today, most casting and splinting is performed by front-line practitioners in the emergency department or by casting technicians. Current residents and fellows in orthopedics, emergency medicine, and primary care specialties are not being exposed to proper techniques, and the accumulated wisdom of generations of orthopedists is in danger of being lost. With this handbook, we hope to catalog the wisdom of our teachers, save the reader from the agony of our mistakes, and prevent patients from being subjected to casts and splints that cause more problems than they solve.

This book is meant for any practitioner who deals with injuries of the musculoskeletal system. For the young practitioner or an older dog trying to pick up new tricks, we recommend reading the general knowledge portions of each section to familiarize yourself with the principles and equipment of musculoskeletal care. What follows are step-by-step, cookbook-style instructions and photographs to guide you through all but the most challenging techniques. Some procedures, as indicated in the text, carry greater risks and are therefore recommended for more experienced practitioners. Happy casting.

Stephen R. Thompson

Dan A. Zlotolow

Although we have worked to ensure the techniques presented here are accurate, we welcome any corrections, suggestions, alternative techniques, or tips you may have. Please email us at thompsonorthopod@gmail.com.

Figure Credits

Contents

PART 1

ANALGESIA

Chapter 1

Basic Principles of Analgesia

Review of Local Anesthetics

1. The two most commonly used local anesthetics are lidocaine (Xylocaine) and bupivacaine (Marcaine, Sensorcaine) (Table 1-1).
   a. Recent studies have suggested that bupivacaine may be toxic to chondrocytes.
   b. Ropivacaine (Naropin) has been found to be significantly less toxic to chondrocytes.
   c. Whenever possible, ropivacaine should be used instead of bupivacaine when performing an intraarticular injection. Unfortunately, ropivacaine is not routinely available in hospital emergency departments.
2. Epinephrine is a vasoconstrictor and is often added to the local anesthetic.
   a. Epinephrine improves onset of action, decreases drug uptake, and prolongs action.
   b. An epinephrine concentration of 1:200,000 is typically used.
   c. Because it is a vasoconstrictor, epinephrine should not be used in the distal extremities. The following well-known mnemonic is often used to recall the areas where epinephrine should not be used: nose, hose (penis), digits, toes.

Types of Local Orthopaedic Analgesia

1. In general, three different techniques are used to achieve local analgesia:
   a. Intra-articular injection
   b. Hematoma block
      (1) A hematoma block involves injection of anesthetic directly into the fracture hematoma.
   c. Nerve block
      (1) A nerve block may be of a specific nerve or of a group of nerves crossing a joint.
      (2) For example, a "wrist block" involves nerve blocks of the radial, median, and ulnar nerves.
2. Regional analgesia also may be established via a Bier block.
   a. A Bier block is accomplished via intravenous injection of a local anesthetic into an extremity with a double raised tourniquet to prevent systemic administration of the anesthetic.
   b. Although it can be useful, a Bier block has the potential for catastrophic complications if the tourniquet fails; thus this procedure should be performed by anesthesiologists familiar with this technique.

TABLE 1-1

LOCAL ANESTHETICS

	Maximum Dosage Concentration	Maximum Dosage Amount	Time Until Effective	Analgesic Action Time	Suggested Use	Comments
Lidocaine	5 mg/kg without epinephrine 7 mg/kg with epinephrine	1% concentration without epinephrine 30-kg child: 15 mL 70-kg adult: 35 mL	2-5 min	45 min-2 h	Short-acting analgesia for 10- to 20-min procedure	Can cause vasodilation if not used with epinephrine
Bupivacaine	1.5 mg/kg without epinephrine 3 mg/kg with epinephrine	0.5% concentration without epinephrine 30-kg child: 9 mL 70-kg adult: 21 mL	10-30 min	3-6 h	Procedure >20 min	Avoid use in intra-articular injection if possible
Ropivacaine	3 mg/kg without epinephrine Not used with epinephrine	0.75% concentration 30-kg child: 12 mL 70-kg adult: 28 mL	7-20 min	2-5 h	Procedure >20 min; safer for use in pediatric population than bupivacaine	Less cardiotoxic than bupivacaine; strong intrinsic vasoconstrictive properties

INDICATIONS FOR USE

1. Intraarticular injection of anesthetic is most commonly used for reduction of ankle fractures.
2. A hematoma block is commonly used for reduction of a variety of fractures and is most often used for a distal radius fracture. Hematoma blocks are performed when selective nerve blocks would not offer adequate analgesia.
3. A nerve block is commonly used for reduction of hand fractures and treatment of soft tissue injuries of the hand.

PRECAUTIONS

1. Unintended intravascular injection of a local anesthetic has the potential to be life-threatening.
2. When injecting an anesthetic, repeated aspiration should be performed to ensure that the needle tip is not intravascular. Use of this technique does not completely exclude the possibility of intravascular injection.
3. Signs and symptoms of intoxication due to local anesthetics are described in Table 1-2.
4. Intraneural injection also should be avoided.
   a. If a needle is inserted and immediate paresthesias are felt by the patient, it is likely that the needle is intraneural.
   b. When it appears that the needle is intraneural, the needle should be withdrawn slightly until the paresthesias are resolved.

PEARLS

1. Sometimes it is useful to spray ethyl chloride (Cryogesic), a topical anesthetic, on the skin overlying the injection site immediately before inserting the needle.
   a. Ethyl chloride should be applied *immediately before* injection because its effects last a very short time.
   b. There is some debate regarding whether ethyl chloride has antimicrobial activity, rendering it acceptable for use on sterilized skin.
2. Palpation of landmarks before beginning the procedure is advisable. Do not hesitate to use a skin pen to mark landmarks or injection sites.

TABLE 1-2
SIGNS AND SYMPTOMS OF INTOXICATION DUE TO LOCAL ANESTHETICS

	Central Nervous System	Cardiovascular System
Mild	Lightheadedness, tingling of lips, tinnitus, tongue paresthesias	Palpitations, tachycardia, hypertension, dry mouth
Moderate	Speech and visual disturbances, confusion, twitching	Arrhythmias, tachycardia, hypotension, cyanosis
Severe	Seizures, flaccidity, coma	Bradycardia and hypotension, ventricular fibrillation

3. Different persons use different techniques for skin preparation.
   a. We prefer using chlorhexidine, which is commercially available in 3-mL applicators.
   b. Alcohol is an alternative skin preparation solution. However, more than one alcohol wipe should be used because one wipe typically contains insufficient alcohol to prepare the skin.
4. The practice of wearing one sterile glove on the nondominant arm is useful because it allows continued palpation of landmarks after the skin has been prepared. This practice also prevents confusion regarding which hand is sterile.

BASIC TECHNIQUE

The basic technique for all procedures is:
1. Prepare anesthetic
2. Palpate landmarks
3. Prepare skin with antiseptic solution
4. Numb skin with ethyl chloride (if desired)
5. Inject anesthetic
6. Place sterile bandage (if desired)

Chapter 2
Hematoma Block

OVERVIEW

1. A hematoma block may be performed anywhere an acute fracture is present.
2. Typically, hematoma blocks are performed in regions where selective nerve blocks or regional blocks are impractical to perform.
3. Hematoma blocks function on the principle that a fracture hematoma surrounds a fracture site.
   a. The fracture hematoma acts as a fluid medium; thus injection of anesthetic into the hematoma results in diffusion of the anesthetic around the fracture site.
   b. Diffusion of the anesthetic around the fracture site results in effective regional anesthesia.

INDICATIONS FOR USE

1. Hematoma blocks are most commonly used for closed reduction of a distal radius fracture.
2. Any diaphyseal or metaphyseal fracture is amenable to a hematoma block.

PRECAUTIONS

1. Hematoma blocks should not be used in patients with broken or tenuous skin overlying the fracture site.
2. Hematoma blocks typically are ineffective in open fractures.

PEARLS

1. A combination of lidocaine and bupivacaine is used to provide both immediate and lasting analgesia. Use of bupivacaine is not mandatory, but fracture reductions are painful, and the use of a long-acting analgesic facilitates recovery in the postreduction period.
2. The injection site can be reasonably approximated with use of palpation and radiographs. Because the periosteum is extremely sensitive, the practice of "walking" the needle down the bone until the fracture site is reached should be avoided.
3. Most patients present for treatment several hours after the initial injury occurred and the fracture hematoma has started to organize. Thus most fracture hematomas cannot be aspirated, and typically no flashback of hematoma is seen in the syringe.
4. A hematoma block typically requires 5 to 10 minutes to become fully effective.

EQUIPMENT

1. Antiseptic: Chlorhexidine prep stick or alcohol-soaked gauze
2. Syringe: 10-mL syringe
3. Needle:
    a. Large-bore, blunt-tipped, drawing-up needle
    b. 1-inch, 22-gauge needle
4. Anesthetic (for a typical adult):
    a. Lidocaine: 5 mL of 2%
    b. Bupivacaine: 5 mL of 0.5%
5. Sterile gloves
6. 4 × 4 inch gauze

BASIC TECHNIQUE

1. Patient positioning:
    a. The extremity should be positioned on a hard surface.
    b. If a distal radius fracture hematoma is being injected, the hematoma block can be performed before or after setting traction.
2. Landmarks:
    a. Fracture site on radiograph
    b. Area of swelling and/or deformity
3. Steps:
    a. Prepare anesthetic
    b. Palpate landmarks
    c. Prepare skin with antiseptic solution
    d. Numb skin with ethyl chloride
    e. Inject anesthetic
    f. Place sterile bandage over injection site (if desired)

DETAILED TECHNIQUE

1. Prepare the anesthetic by drawing up 5 mL of lidocaine and 5 mL of bupivacaine (or age-appropriate lower dose).
2. Palpate landmarks (Figure 2-1):
    a. Use the radiograph to predetermine a soft tissue landmark that can be used as a guide for the precise fracture location.
    b. The deformity or a step-off may be palpable.
3. Prepare the skin with an antiseptic solution. This step may need to be performed several times if the patient's skin is particularly soiled.
4. Numb the skin with ethyl chloride (if desired).
5. Inject the anesthetic (Figure 2-2):
    a. Enter the skin directly over the fracture.
    b. Aspirate the needle while advancing it to avoid intravascular placement of anesthetic. Return of very dark blood suggests that the hematoma has been reached.

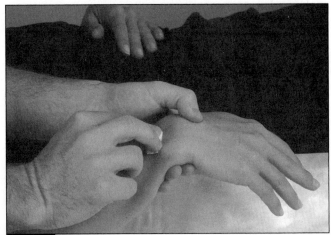

FIGURE 2-1

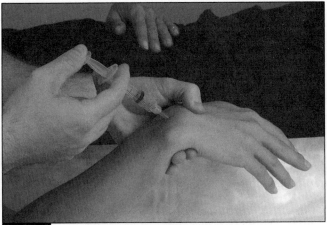

FIGURE 2-2

    c. Inject the anesthetic while being vigilant for any warning signs of intravascular injection.
6. Remove the needle and apply pressure with a gauze bandage.
7. Place a sterile bandage over the injection site if desired.

Chapter 3
Elbow Block

OVERVIEW

The following five nerves are involved in an elbow block: radial, median, ulnar, medial antebrachial cutaneous, and lateral antebrachial cutaneous.
1. The radial and lateral antebrachial cutaneous nerves typically are blocked at the same time because of their proximity to one another.
2. The ulnar and medial antebrachial cutaneous nerves typically are blocked at the same time because of their proximity to one another.

INDICATIONS FOR USE

A complete elbow block can be used when soft tissue procedures that cross dermatomal boundaries are performed.

PRECAUTIONS

Intravascular and intranervous injection is of particular concern when injecting anesthetic around the elbow.

PEARLS

1. The **M**edian nerve lies **M**edial to the brachial artery.
2. To remember the order from lateral to medial, use the mnemonic "**B**reak **R**ight **T**hrough **B**oth **M**ilitary **P**olice" for **B**rachioradialis, **R**adial nerve, biceps **T**endon, **B**rachial artery, **M**edian nerve, and **P**ronator teres.

EQUIPMENT

1. Antiseptic: Chlorhexidine prep stick or alcohol-soaked gauze
2. Syringe: 3×10 mL syringe
3. Needle:
   a. Three large-bore, blunt-tipped, drawing-up needles
   b. Three 1½-inch 25-gauge needles
4. Anesthetic:
   a. Make sure that the dose of anesthetic is safe for the patient's weight and health status.
   b. Lidocaine: 15 mL of 1%
   c. Bupivacaine: 15 mL of 0.5%
      (1) Ulnar and medial antebracheal cutaneous nerves: 10 mL of anesthetic
      (2) Median nerve: 5 mL of anesthetic
      (3) Radial and lateral antebrachial cutaneous nerves: 10 mL of anesthetic
5. Sterile gloves
6. 4×4 inch gauze

BASIC TECHNIQUE

1. Patient positioning: The patient should be seated and a bedside table should be available to position the extremity.
    a. Ulnar nerve and medial antebrachial cutaneous nerve:
        (1) Shoulder at 90 degrees of abduction and external rotation
        (2) Elbow at 90 degrees of flexion
    b. Median nerve:
        (1) Shoulder at 45 degrees of abduction and maximal external rotation
        (2) Elbow extended
    c. Radial and lateral antebrachial cutaneous nerve:
        (1) Shoulder at 45 degrees of abduction and maximal external rotation
        (2) Elbow extended
2. Landmarks:
    a. Ulnar and medial antebrachial cutaneous nerves:
        (1) Medial epicondyle
        (2) Olecranon (a line exists perpendicular to the epicondyle and olecranon)
        (3) Injection of the ulnar nerve is carried out 1 cm proximal to the line between the medial epicondyle and olecranon.
        (4) Injection of the medial antebrachial cutaneous nerve is carried out in a subcutaneous block anterior to the ulnar nerve.
    b. Median nerve:
        (1) Medial and lateral epicondyles: the line between the epicondyles is the *intercondylar line*
        (2) Brachial artery
        (3) Injection of the median nerve is carried out immediately medial to the brachial artery along the intercondylar line.
    c. Radial and lateral antebrachial cutaneous nerve:
        (1) Medial and lateral epicondyles: the line between the epicondyles is the *intercondylar line*
        (2) Biceps tendon
        (3) Injection of the radial and lateral antebrachial cutaneous nerves is carried out 2 cm lateral to the biceps tendon along the intercondylar line.
3. Steps
    a. Block the ulnar and medial antebrachial cutaneous nerves.
    b. Block the median nerve.
    c. Block the radial and lateral antebrachial cutaneous nerve.

DETAILED TECHNIQUE

Prepare Anesthetic

Three syringes should be prepared:

1. Two 10-mL syringes for the radial and lateral antebrachial cutaneous nerves and the ulnar and medial antebracheal cutaneous nerves
2. One 5-mL syringe for the medial nerve

Ulnar and Medial Antebrachial Cutaneous Nerves

1. Position the patient.
2. Palpate landmarks:
   a. Mark the medial epicondyle and the olecranon.
   b. Determine the location of the epicondylar-olecranon line.
   c. Mark the injection site 1 cm proximal to the line.
3. Prepare the skin with an antiseptic solution.
4. Numb the skin with ethyl chloride (if desired).
5. Inject anesthetic (Figure 3-1):
   a. Enter at a 30-degree angle to the skin.
   b. Insert the needle tangentially along the ulnar nerve.
   c. Maintain contact with the patient to ensure that no paresthesias are noted.
   d. Aspirate the needle before injection to ensure that intravascular placement has been avoided.
   e. Inject 5 mL of anesthetic immediately below the skin. Be vigilant for any warning signs of intravascular injection.
   f. Redirect the needle anteriorly and advance subcutaneously to the hilt (Figure 3-2).
   g. Withdraw the needle while injecting the remaining 5 mL of anesthetic.
6. Place a sterile bandage over the injection site.

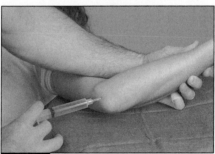
FIGURE 3-1

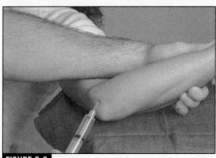
FIGURE 3-2

Median Nerve

1. Position the patient.
2. Palpate landmarks:
   a. Feel the medial and lateral epicondyles.
   b. Mark the intercondylar line.
   c. Palpate the brachial artery.
   d. Mark the injection site immediately medial to the brachial artery.
3. Prepare the skin with an antiseptic solution.
4. Numb the skin with ethyl chloride (if desired).
5. Inject anesthetic (Figure 3-3):
   a. Enter the skin directly over the nerve.
   b. Insert the needle; aim slightly medially.
   c. Maintain contact with the patient to ensure that no paresthesias are noted.
   d. Aspirate the needle before injection to ensure that intravascular placement has been avoided.
   e. Inject 3 to 5 mL of anesthetic at a depth of 0.5 to 1 cm. Be vigilant for any warning signs of intravascular injection.
6. Place a sterile bandage over the injection site.

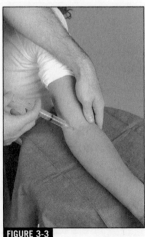

FIGURE 3-3

Radial and Lateral Antebrachial Cutaneous Nerves

1. Position the patient.
2. Palpate landmarks:
   a. Feel the medial and lateral epicondyles.
   b. Mark the intercondylar line.
   c. Palpate the biceps tendon.
   d. Mark the injection site 2 cm lateral to the biceps tendon along the intercondylar line.
3. Prepare the skin with an antiseptic solution.

4. Numb the skin with ethyl chloride (if desired).
5. Inject anesthetic (Figure 3-4):
    a. Enter the skin directly over the nerve.
    b. Insert the needle; aim slightly laterally and proximally toward the lateral epicondyle.
    c. Maintain contact with the patient to determine if paresthesias are noted.
        (1) If paresthesias are elicited, withdraw the needle very slightly.
        (2) If paresthesias are not elicited, advance the needle to bone.
    d. Aspirate the needle before injection to ensure that intravascular placement has been avoided.
    e. Inject 5 mL of anesthetic at a depth determined by the presence or absence of paresthesias. Be vigilant for any warning signs of intravascular injection.
    f. Slowly withdraw the needle until it is in a subcutaneous position.
    g. Inject 5 mL of anesthetic in a fan-shaped pattern.
6. Place a sterile bandage over the injection site.

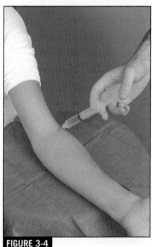

FIGURE 3-4

Chapter 4
Wrist Block

OVERVIEW

The following three nerves are involved in an wrist block: radial, median, and ulnar.

1. The ulnar nerve has a dorsal sensory branch that arises 5 cm proximal to the wrist crease.
2. Two techniques can be used to block the ulnar nerve.
   a. Proximal block:
      (1) A proximal block anesthetizes the ulnar nerve approximately 6 cm proximal to the wrist crease.
      (2) In most cases, a proximal block will block both branches.
      (3) Variable anatomy is always a risk.
   b. Distal block:
      (1) The ulnar nerve is anesthetized near the wrist crease and the injection of anesthetic is directed both volarly to anesthetize the ulnar nerve and dorsally to anesthetize the dorsal cutaneous branch.
      (2) The distal block technique ensures that both branches are consistently blocked.
      (3) The distal block is the favored technique.

INDICATIONS FOR USE

1. A complete wrist block can be used when soft tissue procedures that cross dermatomal boundaries are performed.
2. Selective nerve blocks:
   a. Ulnar: Reduction of fractures about the small finger (particularly boxer's fractures) and ulnar-sided soft tissue concerns
   b. Median: Fingertip injuries to the index and long fingers
   c. Radial: Reduction of fractures about the thumb and dorsal hand soft tissue concerns

PRECAUTIONS

1. Intravascular injection is of particular concern when injecting anesthetic around the wrist.
2. Use of epinephrine should be avoided in wrist blocks.

PEARLS

1. Asking the patient to make a fist can aid in palpation of anatomic landmarks.
2. When injecting anesthetic near the ulnar nerve, look for a fullness in the area radial to the flexor carpi ulnaris (FCU) tendon to confirm correct placement.

EQUIPMENT

1. Antiseptic: Chlorhexidine prep stick or alcohol-soaked gauze
2. Syringe: Three 10-mL syringes
3. Needle:
    a. Large-bore, blunt-tipped, drawing-up needles
    b. 1-inch, 25-gauge needle
4. Anesthetic (for a typical adult):
    a. Lidocaine: 15 mL of 1%
    b. Bupivacaine: 15 mL of 0.5%
        (1) Ulnar nerve: 8 to 10 mL of anesthetic
        (2) Median nerve: 3 to 5 mL of anesthetic
        (3) Radial nerve: 5 to 8 mL of anesthetic
5. Sterile gloves
6. 4 × 4 inch gauze

BASIC TECHNIQUE

1. Patient positioning:
    a. The patient should be seated and a bedside table should be available to position the extremity.
    b. For median and ulnar nerve blocks, lay the extremity on a bedside table with the elbow extended and the hand supinated.
    c. For radial nerve blocks, lay the extremity on a bedside table with the elbow extended and the hand pronated.
2. Landmarks:
    a. Ulnar nerve:
        (1) FCU tendon
        (2) Ulnar styloid
        (3) Injection of the ulnar nerve is carried out 0.5 cm proximal to the ulnar styloid under the FCU tendon.
    b. Median nerve:
        (1) Palmaris longus tendon
        (2) Flexor carpi radialis (FCR) tendon
            (a) The palmaris longus tendon is the more prominent and more medial tendon.
            (b) Be aware that the palmaris longus is absent in about 10% to 20% of patients. If only one tendon can be palpated, it is the FCR tendon.
        (3) Wrist crease
        (4) Injection of the median nerve is carried out 2 cm proximal to the wrist crease between the FCR and palmaris longus tendons.
    c. Radial nerve:
        (1) Radial styloid
3. Steps:
    a. Block the ulnar nerve.
    b. Block the median nerve.
    c. Block the radial and lateral antebrachial cutaneous nerves.

Prepare the anesthetic; three 10-mL syringes should be prepared.

Ulnar Nerve

1. Position the patient and palpate landmarks:
   a. Palpate the FCU tendon (Figure 4-1) and ulnar styloid.
   b. Mark the FCU tendon and ulnar styloid.
   c. Mark the injection site 0.5 cm proximal to the ulnar styloid under the FCU tendon.
2. Prepare the skin with an antiseptic solution.
3. Numb the skin with ethyl chloride (if desired).
4. Inject the anesthetic (Figure 4-2).
   a. Insert the needle at a 90-degree angle to the skin under the FCU tendon.

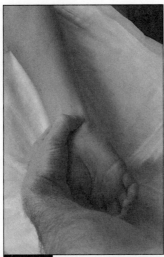

FIGURE 4-1

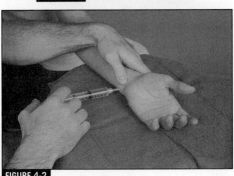

FIGURE 4-2

   b. Maintain patient contact to ensure no paresthesias are noted.
   c. Aspirate the needle before injection to ensure that intravascular placement has been avoided.
   d. Advance the needle 0.5 to 1 cm.
   e. Inject 3 to 5 mL of anesthetic. Be vigilant for any warning signs of intravascular injection. Withdraw the needle to a subcutaneous position.
   f. Redirect the needle dorsally and advance the length of the needle to cover the dorsal sensory branch of the ulnar nerve (Figure 4-3).
   g. Withdraw the needle slowly while injecting 2 to 3 mL of anesthetic subcutaneously.
5. Place a sterile bandage over the injection site.

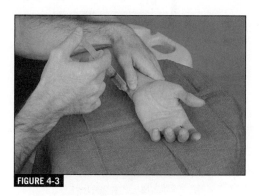

FIGURE 4-3

Median Nerve
1. Position the patient.
2. Palpate landmarks:
   a. Palpate the FCR tendon and palmaris longus.
   b. Mark the FCR tendon and palmaris longus.
   c. Mark the injection site at the wrist crease just ulnar to the palmaris longus.
3. Prepare the skin with an antiseptic solution.
4. Numb the skin with ethyl chloride (if desired).

5. Inject anesthetic:
   a. Enter at a 45-degree angle to the skin (Figure 4-4).
   b. Immediately inject 1 to 2 mL of anesthetic subcutaneously to block the palmar cutaneous branch (supplying the skin of the central palm).
   c. Maintain contact with the patient to ensure no paresthesias are noted.
   d. Advance the needle until the fascia has been penetrated (a click or pop sometimes can be felt) or the needle contacts bone. If the needle contacts bone, withdraw 2 to 3 mm.
   e. Inject 3 to 5 mL of anesthetic.
6. Place a sterile bandage over the injection site.

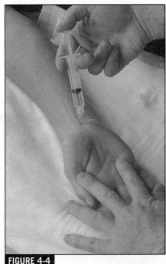

FIGURE 4-4

Radial Nerve

1. Position the patient.
2. Palpate landmarks:
   a. Feel the radial styloid.
   b. Mark the injection site 0.5 cm proximal to the radial styloid and slightly dorsal.

3. Prepare the skin with an antiseptic solution.
4. Numb the skin with ethyl chloride (if desired).
5. Inject anesthetic (Figures 4-5 and 4-6):
    a. Enter at a 90-degree angle to the skin.
    b. Insert the needle, aimed in a volar direction.
    c. Maintain contact with the patient to determine if paresthesias are noted.
    d. Aspirate the needle before injection to ensure that intravascular placement has been avoided.
    e. Advance the needle its full length.
    f. Inject 5 mL of anesthetic. Be vigilant for any warning signs of intravascular injection.
    g. Slowly withdraw the needle until it is in a subcutaneous position.
    h. Redirect the needle dorsally.
    i. Advance the needle subcutaneously along the dorsum of the wrist.
    j. Inject 5 mL of anesthetic in a ring fashion.
6. Place a sterile bandage over the injection site.

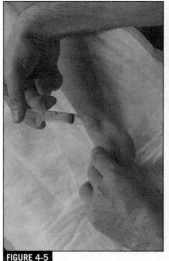

FIGURE 4-5

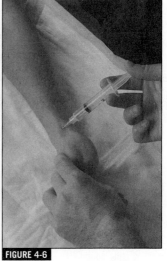

FIGURE 4-6

Chapter 5
Digital Block

OVERVIEW

1. Two techniques can be used to perform a digital block:
   a. Tendon sheath injection
   b. Web space injection
2. The web space injection technique is more painful but provides a complete digital block more reliably.

INDICATIONS FOR USE

A digital block is used for soft tissue injuries about the finger distal to the proximal interphalangeal joint.

PRECAUTIONS

1. Warnings not to use epinephrine in a digit are based on misinterpretations of invalidated data.
2. Do not use a digital block if the metacarpophalangeal (MP) joint is surrounded by infection.

PEARLS

When performing a tendon sheath injection, the dorsal block can be enhanced by skirting the tendon sheath on either side and injecting on the dorsum of the hand.

EQUIPMENT

1. Antiseptic: Chlorhexidine prep stick or alcohol-soaked gauze
2. Syringe: 10-mL syringe
3. Needle:
   a. Large-bore, blunt-tipped, drawing-up needle
   b. 1½-inch, 25-gauge needle
4. Anesthetic (for a typical adult):
   a. Lidocaine: 5 mL of 2%
   b. Bupivacaine: 5 mL of 0.5%
5. Sterile gloves
6. 4 × 4 inch gauze

BASIC TECHNIQUE

1. Patient positioning: Place the hand on a bedside table with the arm in pronation.
2. Landmarks:
   a. Web space on either side of the affected digit or tendon sheath
   b. The digital nerves are injected on either side of the affected digit.
3. Steps:
   a. Position the patient.
   b. Prepare the anesthetic.
   c. Palpate landmarks.
   d. Prepare the skin with an antiseptic solution.
   e. Numb the skin with ethyl chloride (if desired).
   f. Inject anesthetic:
      (1) Inject anesthetic on both sides for a web space block.
      (2) Inject anesthetic on the volar tendon sheath and incorporate dorsal skin.
   g. Place a sterile bandage over the injection site.

DETAILED TECHNIQUE

1. Position the patient.
2. Prepare the anesthetic. A single 10-mL syringe is required.
3. Palpate landmarks.
4. Prepare the skin with an antiseptic solution.
5. Numb the skin with ethyl chloride (if desired).
6. Inject anesthetic (web space injection):
   a. Enter from the dorsal aspect at a 90-degree angle to the skin.
   b. Insert the needle, aiming in a volar direction.
   c. Maintain patient contact to note any paresthesias.
   d. Aspirate the needle before injection to ensure that intravascular placement has been avoided.
   e. Advance the needle volarly until it is almost subcutaneous.
   f. Inject 2 mL of anesthetic. Be vigilant for any warning signs of intravascular injection.
   g. Slowly withdraw the needle. Repeatedly aspirate and then inject another 1 mL as the needle is withdrawn.
   h. Repeat the injection on the other side of the digit.

7. Inject anesthetic (tendon sheath injection):
   a. Enter from the volar aspect just proximal to the MP joint at a 90-degree angle to the skin for the thumb (Figure 5-1) and fingers (Figure 5-2).
   b. Insert the needle, aiming at the flexor sheath in a dorsal direction.
   c. Maintain patient contact to note any paresthesias.
   d. Aspirate the needle before injection to ensure that intravascular placement has been avoided.
   e. Advance the needle until it contacts the tendon sheath.
   f. Inject 5 mL of anesthetic. Be vigilant for any warning signs of intravascular injection.
   g. Slowly withdraw the needle to the level of the subcutaneous tissue.

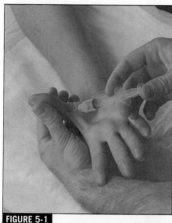
FIGURE 5-1

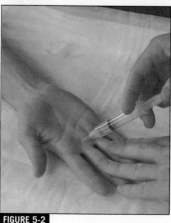
FIGURE 5-2

    h. Redirect the needle to skirt the flexor sheath on either side and advance into the dorsum of the hand (Figure 5-3). Repeatedly aspirate the needle and then inject another 2.5 mL.

    i. Repeat the injection on other side of the flexor sheath.

8. Place a sterile bandage over the injection site.

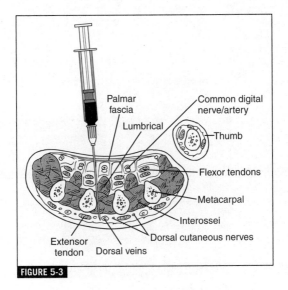

FIGURE 5-3

Chapter 6
Ankle Block

OVERVIEW

1. The following five nerves are involved in an ankle block: posterior tibial, superficial peroneal, deep peroneal, saphenous, and sural.
2. The posterior tibial and deep peroneal nerves are deep to the fascia, whereas the remainder of the nerves are superficial.

INDICATIONS FOR USE

1. Foot fracture reduction
2. Soft tissue injuries about the foot

PRECAUTIONS

1. Avoid intravascular and intraneural injections.
2. Do not use an ankle block for fractures of the ankle.

PEARLS

1. The posterior tibial and deep peroneal nerve blocks should be performed first, because these nerves are deep to the fascia. Attempting to block the superficial nerves first will result in subcutaneous injection of anesthetic that may distort local anatomy.
2. The superficial nerves require only a subcutaneous injection of anesthetic.

EQUIPMENT

1. Antiseptic: Chlorhexidine prep stick or alcohol-soaked gauze
2. Syringe: Three 10-mL syringes
3. Needle:
   a. Large-bore, blunt-tipped, drawing-up needle
   b. 1½-inch, 25-gauge needle
4. Anesthetic:
   a. Lidocaine: 15 mL of 2%
   b. Bupivacaine: 15 mL of 0.5%
5. Sterile gloves
6. 4 × 4 inch gauze

BASIC TECHNIQUE

1. Patient positioning:
   a. The patient is supine.
   b. The leg should be positioned either on a footrest or off the edge of the bed.
   c. The posterior aspect of the ankle must be accessible.
2. Landmarks:
   a. Posterior tibial nerve:
      (1) Medial malleolus
      (2) Posterior tibial artery (the nerve is *posterior* to this)
   b. Deep peroneal nerve:
      (1) Medial and lateral malleoli (the line connecting the two malleoli is the *intermalleolar line*)
      (2) Extensor hallucis longus (EHL) tendon
      (3) Extensor digitorum longus (EDL) tendon
      (4) Anterior tibial artery (dorsalis pedis) (the nerve is immediately *lateral* to the artery)
   c. Superficial peroneal nerve: Lateral malleolus
   d. Saphenous nerve: Medial malleolus
   e. Sural nerve:
      (1) Lateral malleolus
      (2) Lateral border of Achilles tendon
      (3) Calcaneus
3. Steps:
   a. Block the posterior tibial nerve.
   b. Block the deep peroneal nerve.
   c. Block the superficial peroneal nerve.
   d. Block the saphenous nerve.
   e. Block the sural nerve.

DETAILED TECHNIQUE

Prepare the anesthetic. Three syringes should be prepared.

Posterior Tibial Nerve

1. Position the patient.
2. Palpate landmarks:
   a. Palpate the medial malleolus and posterior tibial artery.
   b. Mark the medial malleolus and posterior tibial artery, if desired.
   c. Mark the injection site immediately posterior to the tibial artery at the level of the medial malleolus.
3. Prepare the skin with an antiseptic solution.
4. Numb the skin with ethyl chloride (if desired).
5. Inject anesthetic (Figure 6-1):
   a. Enter at a 90-degree angle to the skin.
   b. Maintain patient contact to note any paresthesias.
   c. Aspirate the needle before injection to ensure that intravascular placement has been avoided.
   d. Advance the needle until contact is made with the bone.
   e. Withdraw the needle 1 to 2 mm.
   f. Inject 3 to 5 mL of anesthetic. Be vigilant for any warning signs of intravascular injection.
   g. Use a fan technique to block cutaneous branches or anomalous anatomic branches.
      (1) Withdraw the needle to a subcutaneous position.
      (2) Redirect anteriorly and advance 0.5 cm.
      (3) Inject 2 mL of anesthetic.
      (4) Withdraw the needle to a subcutaneous position.
      (5) Redirect posteriorly and advance 0.5 cm.
      (6) Inject 2 mL of anesthetic.
6. Place a sterile bandage over the injection site.

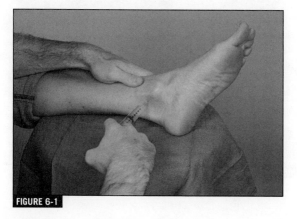

FIGURE 6-1

Deep Peroneal Nerve

1. Position the patient.
2. Palpate landmarks:
   a. Palpate the medial and lateral malleoli. Identify and mark the intermalleolar line.
   b. Palpate the EHL tendon by having the patient dorsiflex the hallux.
   c. Palpate the EDL tendon by having the patient dorsiflex the lesser toes.
   d. Palpate the dorsalis pedis artery.
   e. Mark these four structures.
   f. Mark the injection site between the EDL and EHL tendons and 2 cm distal to the intermalleolar line. This position is on the lateral border of the dorsalis pedis artery.
3. Prepare the skin with an antiseptic solution.
4. Numb the skin with ethyl chloride (if desired).
5. Inject anesthetic (Figure 6-2):
   a. Enter at a 60-degree angle to the skin.
   b. Maintain contact with the patient to ensure that no paresthesias are noted.
   c. Aspirate the needle before injection to ensure that intravascular placement has been avoided.
   d. Advance the needle until contact is made with the bone.
   e. Withdraw the needle 1 to 2 mm.
   f. Inject 5 mL of anesthetic. Be vigilant for any warning signs of intravascular injection.
6. Place a sterile bandage over the injection site.

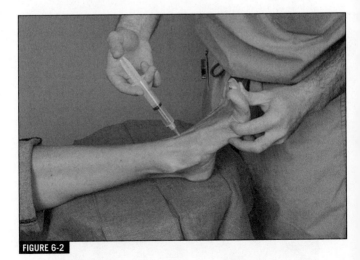

FIGURE 6-2

Superficial Peroneal Nerve/Sural Nerve

1. Position the patient.
2. Palpate landmarks (Figure 6-3):
   a. Feel the lateral malleolus.
   b. Mark the injection site the breadth of two fingers distal to the tip of the lateral malleolus.
3. Prepare the skin with an antiseptic solution.
4. Numb the skin with ethyl chloride (if desired).
5. Inject the anesthetic in a ring-type block (Figure 6-4).
   a. Enter at a 45-degree angle to the skin.
   b. Insert the needle, aiming it in a lateral direction.
   c. Maintain contact with the patient to determine if paresthesias are noted.
   d. Aspirate the needle before injection to ensure that intravascular placement has been avoided.
   e. Advance the needle subcutaneously.
   f. Inject 5 mL of anesthetic from the lateral to medial aspect while withdrawing the needle. Be vigilant for any warning signs of intravascular injection.
6. Place a sterile bandage over the injection site.

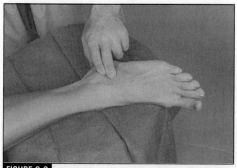

FIGURE 6-3

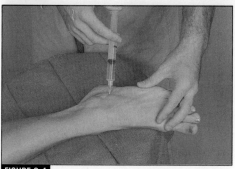

FIGURE 6-4

Saphenous Nerve

1. Position the patient.
2. Palpate landmarks:
   a. Feel the medial malleolus.
   b. Mark the injection site the breadth of two fingers proximal to the tip of the medial malleolus and the breadth of one finger anterior.
3. Prepare the skin with an antiseptic solution.
4. Numb the skin with ethyl chloride (if desired).
5. Inject the anesthetic in a ring-type block (Figure 6-5).
   a. Enter at a 45-degree angle to the skin.
   b. Insert the needle, aiming it posteriorly and distally.
   c. Maintain contact with the patient to determine if paresthesias are noted.
   d. Aspirate the needle before injection to ensure that intravascular placement has been avoided.
   e. Advance the needle subcutaneously.
   f. Inject 2 to 3 mL of anesthetic from the posterior to anterior aspect while withdrawing the needle. Be vigilant for any warning signs of intravascular injection.
6. Place a sterile bandage over the injection site.

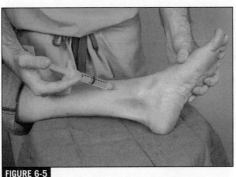

FIGURE 6-5

Chapter 7
Intra-articular Ankle Block

OVERVIEW

When performing an intra-articular ankle block, an anterolateral approach is preferred.

INDICATIONS FOR USE

The intra-articular ankle block is used for ankle fracture reduction.

PRECAUTIONS

1. Use of the lateral malleolus as a landmark helps prevent damage to the dorsal cutaneous nerve.
2. In patients with significant swelling, tendinous structures are difficult to palpate.

PEARLS

1. A topical anesthetic with ethyl chloride may be used to reduce patient discomfort.
2. Positioning the ankle in slight plantarflexion provides easier access to the joint.

EQUIPMENT

1. Antiseptic: Chlorhexidine prep stick
2. Syringe: 10-mL syringe
3. Anesthetic:
   a. Lidocaine: 5 mL of 2%
   b. Bupivacaine: 5 mL of 0.5%
4. Needle: 1½-inch, 22-gauge needle
5. Sterile gloves
6. 4 × 4 inch gauze

BASIC TECHNIQUE

1. The patient should be supine with the ankle in slight plantarflexion.
2. Landmarks:
   a. Lateral malleolus
   b. Peroneus tertius tendon
      (1) The site of entry is 2.5 cm proximal and 1.3 cm anterior to the tip of the lateral malleolus.
      (2) This site of entry is immediately lateral to the peroneus tertius tendon.
3. Steps:
   a. Position the patient.
   b. Palpate landmarks.

c. Prepare the skin with an antiseptic solution.
d. Place sterile drapes around the ankle.
e. Administer a topical anesthetic, if desired.
f. Inject anesthetic into the joint.
g. Place a sterile bandage over the injection site.

DETAILED TECHNIQUE

1. Position the patient so he or she is supine with the ankle in slight plantarflexion.
2. Palpate landmarks:
   a. Feel the most distal aspect of the lateral malleolus.
   b. The site of entry is slightly more than the breadth of one finger proximal and half the breadth of a finger anterior.
   c. Mark this site.
3. Prepare the skin with an antiseptic solution. Perform a wide preparation.
4. Place sterile drapes around the ankle. Drape out proximally, distally, and laterally.
5. Administer a topical anesthetic, if desired.
6. Inject anesthetic into the joint (Figure 7-1):
   a. Enter at a 60-degree angle to the skin.
   b. Insert the needle in a posterior and medial direction.
   c. Advance 0.5 to 1 cm to enter the joint.
   d. Inject the anesthetic.
7. Place a sterile bandage over the injection site.

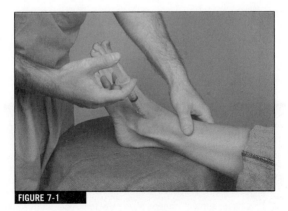

FIGURE 7-1

PART 2

REDUCTION MANEUVERS

Chapter 8

Basic Principles of Reduction Maneuvers

THE THREE-POINT PRINCIPLE

1. Diaphyseal fractures (Figure 8-1, *A*):
   a. The primary reductive force should be applied against the apex of the fracture.
   b. Counterforce applied in the opposite direction both proximal and distal to the apex stabilizes the limb.
2. Metaphyseal/epiphyseal fractures (Figure 8-1, *B*):
   a. The primary reductive force should be applied just distal to the fracture.
   b. Counterforce should be applied in the opposite direction just proximal to the fracture and in the same direction as the primary force at the proximal end of the bone.

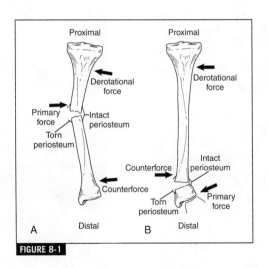

FIGURE 8-1

35

EXAGGERATING THE DEFORMITY

1. Indications for reduction by exaggerating the deformity:
   a. Fully displaced fractures with an intact periosteal hinge (typically in children) and bayonet apposition (Figure 8-2)
   b. Fracture fragments that will not disengage with traction and/or direct reduction maneuvers (Figure 8-3)
   c. Rarely indicated for diaphyseal fractures
2. The principle of this reduction method is to:
   a. Disengage the fracture fragments (Figure 8-4)
   b. Allow direct reduction methods to succeed (Figure 8-5)

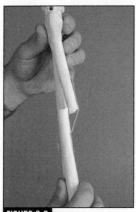

FIGURE 8-2

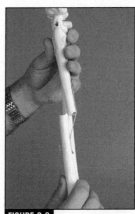

FIGURE 8-3

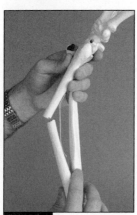

FIGURE 8-4

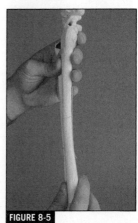

FIGURE 8-5

3. Technique:
    a. Begin with manually applied traction and countertraction.
    b. Place a thumb or two just proximal to the fracture on the side opposite the apex as a fulcrum.
    c. Apply a point of counterforce proximal to the fracture on the side of the apex.
    d. Exaggerate the deformity by accentuating the apex so that the angulation of the fracture exceeds 90 degrees.
    e. Using the thumb(s), push distalward, moving the fulcrum more distal.
    f. Correct the deformity and reduce the fracture.

THE VALUE OF TRACTION

1. Overcoming muscle force:
    a. The skeleton counteracts the contractile forces of the muscles.
    b. Muscles pulling against a broken bone will shorten it.
    c. Fractures and muscle injury result in involuntary muscle spasm.
    d. Traction allows the bone to be restored to its proper length by overcoming muscle contraction and spasm.
    e. The amount of traction applied should exceed the amount of muscle spasm.
2. Disimpacting fractures:
    a. Fracture fragments can become locked by interdigitating.
    b. Distraction allows for reduction by translation.
3. Taking advantage of the soft tissue envelope:
    a. Comminuted fractures can be reduced by hydrostatic pressure.
    b. Intact tendons, muscles, and periosteum can directly reduce areas of comminution.

8

4. Applying traction:
   a. Double digit construct:
      (1) Make a loop of gauze with your left hand.
      (2) Place your right thumb and index finger inside the loop in supination (Figure 8-6).
      (3) While holding one side of the gauze taut with the left hand, spread your right index finger and thumb apart, then pronate your right forearm (Figure 8-7).

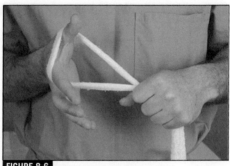

FIGURE 8-6

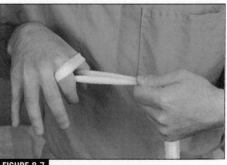

FIGURE 8-7

(4) Your index finger and thumb should now be outside the loop.
(5) Bring the tips of your index finger and thumb together and pull the loops out with your index finger (Figure 8-8).
(6) Place each of the newly formed traction loops around each of the fingers or toes to which traction will be applied (Figure 8-9).
(7) Make sure the transverse limb connecting both traction loops is behind the free end of the gauze (Figure 8-10).
(8) Attach the free end of the gauze to an intravenous line pole or another well-anchored elevation device.

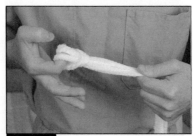

FIGURE 8-8

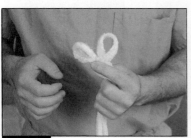

FIGURE 8-9

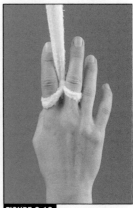

FIGURE 8-10

b. Single digit construct (Figure 8-11):
   (1) Follow the outlined steps for the double digit construct, but place both traction loops around same digit (Figure 8-12).
c. Alternatively, commercially available Chinese finger traps may be used (Figure 8-13).
   (1) We have found that Chinese finger traps are liable to come loose during the application of traction.
   (2) Mastisol or benzoin may be applied to the skin to prevent finger trap migration.

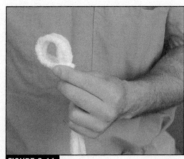

FIGURE 8-11

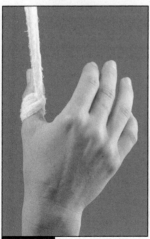

FIGURE 8-12

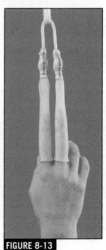

FIGURE 8-13

d. Use commercially available weight trees to attach the weights and provide traction (Figure 8-14).
   (1) If a weight tree is not available:
      (a) Take a 4-foot length of stockinette and securely tie one end.
      (b) Place two 5-lb weights inside the stockinette.
      (c) Securely tie the other end.
      (d) Separate the two weights and place the stockinette over the arm (Figure 8-15).
   (2) If weights are not available, use large intravenous bags (Figure 8-16) in place of the weights and follow the aforementioned procedure.

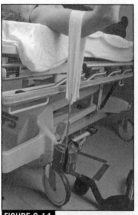

FIGURE 8-14

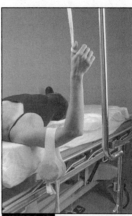

FIGURE 8-15

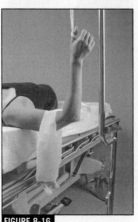

FIGURE 8-16

PHYSEAL INJURIES

1. Reduction of a Salter-Harris fracture (Figure 8-17) should be attempted only after one is skilled with adult fractures and extraphyseal pediatric fractures in that region.
2. A level of anesthesia that will limit muscle spasm and involuntary or voluntary muscle contraction should be attained and may be achieved through one of the following methods:
   a. General anesthesia
   b. Conscious sedation
   c. Dissociative anesthesia (ketamine)
3. The number of reduction attempts should be limited to one or two.
4. Use of excessive force should be avoided.
5. More traction than is typical should be used to fully disengage the fracture before attempting a reduction.
6. Traction should be maintained throughout reduction maneuvers.
7. Repeated and/or forceful reduction attempts may further damage the physis and result in physeal arrest or bar formation.
   a. A consequence may be limited growth or angulation of the limb.
   b. This complication is very difficult to treat.

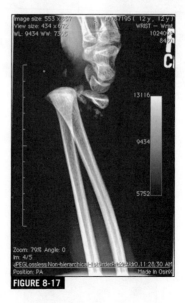

FIGURE 8-17

JOINT REDUCTIONS

1. Principles similar to those of fracture reduction apply to joint reduction.
2. A satisfying "clunk" is usually heard upon successful joint reduction.
3. Soft tissue interposition and buttonholing may preclude joint reduction.

PRECAUTIONS

1. Avoid placing either primary force or counterforce directly over the following potential sites of nerve compression when molding a splint or cast or when obtaining a reduction in plaster:
   a. Axilla
   b. Cubital tunnel
   c. Carpal tunnel
   d. Femoral triangle
   e. Popliteal fossa
   f. Fibular head
   g. Tarsal tunnel
2. Use broad surfaces such as the palm of the hand for the reduction whenever possible to distribute force over a larger area.
3. The exaggeration of deformity technique should be used with caution and only when direct reduction techniques fail. An intact periosteal hinge prevents reduction by direct means but prevents over-reduction and complete destabilization of the fracture.
4. When a fracture fragment or joint is buttonholed through fascia or between two tendons/ligaments, traction will complicate the reduction.
   a. If reduction becomes more difficult with traction, try the reduction without traction.
   b. If all reduction attempts fail, consider soft tissue interposition as a cause, obtain the best reduction possible, and make arrangements for an open reduction in the operating room.

PEARLS

1. If the periosteal hinge is intact, it is nearly impossible to over-reduce the fracture.
2. To correct angulation only, a three-point bend is sufficient.
3. To correct translation only, use traction to disengage the fragments, then apply a correcting force just distal to the fracture as well as a counterforce just proximal to the fracture.
4. To correct rotation, flex the next most distal joint and use the direction of flexion as a guide and a handle to dial in rotation.
5. Use a leg, a knee, or the stretcher to provide counterforce if necessary.

IMPROVISATION

1. When all else fails, develop a clear picture of the fracture in your head and then imagine how you would intuitively reduce it.
2. Each fracture is different, and improvisation is encouraged after standard techniques have failed.

Chapter 9
Shoulder and Elbow Reduction

CLAVICLE FRACTURE

Overview

1. Most clavicle fractures require no reduction.
2. Closed reductions cannot be maintained and should not be attempted.

Indications for Use

1. Minimally displaced clavicle shaft fractures (Figure 9-1)
2. Medial physeal clavicle fractures

Precautions

Do not attempt heroic measures to reduce clavicle fractures.

Pearls

1. Clavicle fractures with more than 1.5 cm of overlap result in long-term disability and should be treated with an open reduction and internal fixation.
2. Fractures that tent the skin can erode through the skin and are unlikely to heal without open reduction and internal fixation.
3. There is no difference in outcome between a figure-of-8 splint and a sling for closed management of clavicle fractures.
4. The sling or figure-of-8 strap should be relatively tight to support the weight of the arm.

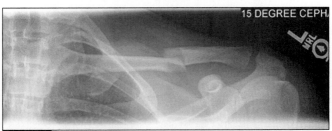

15 DEGREE CEPH.

FIGURE 9-1

Improvisation

If no sling is available, a simple scarf or towel can be used.

Equipment

1. Sling
2. Figure-of-8 strap (alternative)

Basic/Detailed Technique

1. Sling (see Chapter 13)
2. Figure-of-8 strap (see Chapter 13)

ACROMIOCLAVICULAR SEPARATION

Overview

1. Most acromioclavicular (AC) separations require no reduction.
2. Closed reductions cannot be maintained and should not be attempted.

Indications for Use

1. Minimally displaced AC separations (grades 1 to 3) (Figure 9-2)
2. Severely displaced AC separations (grades 4 to 6) (Figure 9-3)

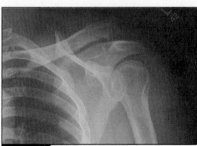

FIGURE 9-2

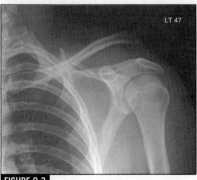

FIGURE 9-3

Precautions

Do not attempt heroic measures to reduce AC separations.

Pearls

1. AC separations with severe displacement or soft tissue interposition (grades 4 to 6) should be reduced surgically on an elective basis.
2. AC separations that tent the skin are unlikely to heal without fixation.
3. The sling should be relatively tight to support the weight of the arm.

Improvisation

If no sling is available, a simple scarf or towel can be used.

Equipment

Sling

Basic/Detailed Technique

Sling (see Chapter 13)

GLENOHUMERAL DISLOCATION

Overview

1. Most glenohumeral dislocations can be reduced in a closed manner.
2. The reduction technique varies according to the direction of dislocation.
3. An axillary or modified axillary view is an essential part of the radiographic series (Figure 9-4)!

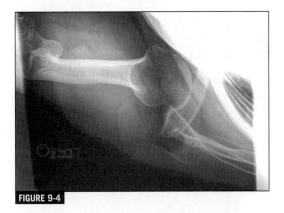

FIGURE 9-4

Indications for Use

1. Anterior glenohumeral dislocation
2. Posterior glenohumeral dislocation
3. Inferior glenohumeral dislocation (luxatio erecta)

Precautions

1. Confirm that no fracture is present on diagnostic films before attempting a reduction. Standard reduction maneuvers can result in a displaced four-part fracture that requires surgical fixation/prosthetic replacement.
2. Confirm that the humeral head is not impacted onto the glenoid (known as a Hill-Sachs lesion) before attempting a reduction (see Figure 9-4). Standard reduction maneuvers can result in a head-splitting fracture.
3. When applying traction, make sure that the force is applied over a broad area; otherwise, a forearm fracture can result.
4. Be aware that some persons may voluntarily initiate a glenohumeral dislocation in an effort to gain access to drugs.
5. Reducing dislocations in persons who present more than a few days after the injury may not be possible, and attempting to do so could result in a fracture; it is preferable not to attempt a reduction and to take the patient to the operating room if simple traction does not succeed in reducing the dislocation.
6. When reducing posterior dislocations, do not externally rotate the humerus until the head is disimpacted from the glenoid or a fracture may result.

Pearls

1. Be patient; the stability of the shoulder is provided largely by a set of small but powerful muscles that must be overcome with gentle sustained traction before a reduction is possible.
2. Gentle internal and external rotation of the shoulder can coax the humerus back in place.
3. For posterior dislocations, stretching the rotator cuff muscles by maximal internal rotation of the shoulder may be necessary.
4. General anesthesia may be required if muscle spasms are not overcome with sedation.
5. External rotation is a better position for immobilization of both anterior and posterior dislocations after reduction, although a gunslinger brace may not be available immediately.
6. The sling or gunslinger brace can be applied loosely for comfort.

Improvisation

When all else fails, try traction at different angles of abduction and extension.

ANTERIOR GLENOHUMERAL DISLOCATION

Equipment

1. Two bed sheets
2. Stretcher
3. Medications for conscious sedation
4. Sling or gunslinger brace (if available)

Basic Technique

1. Patient positioning:
   a. The patient is supine on the stretcher.
   b. The patient's elbow is bent 90 degrees and the forearm is vertical.
   c. The patient's shoulder is abducted 30 to 60 degrees.
   d. A bed sheet is tied around the patient's trunk and to the opposite side of the stretcher.
   e. A bed sheet is tied around your waist and to the patient's forearm.
2. Landmarks:
   a. Acromion
   b. Humeral head
   c. Coracoid
3. Steps:
   a. Position the patient.
   b. Induce sedation.
   c. Tie the bed sheet to the stretcher.
   d. Tie the bed sheet to yourself.
   e. Lean back to apply traction.
   f. Gently externally rotate the shoulder.
   g. Await a clunk as the shoulder reduces.
   h. Place the shoulder in a sling or gunslinger brace.
   i. Obtain postreduction films.

Detailed Technique

1. Position the patient supine on the stretcher.
2. Induce conscious sedation.
3. Prepare traction setup:
   a. Make sure that guard rails are down on the ipsilateral side and up on the contralateral side.
   b. Slide a rolled bed sheet around the patient's trunk under the ipsilateral shoulder and tie it over the contralateral upper corner of the stretcher for countertraction (Figures 9-5 and 9-6).
   c. Tie another rolled bed sheet around your waist, leaving about a foot of slack.

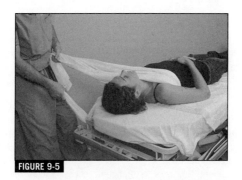

FIGURE 9-5

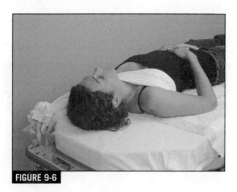

FIGURE 9-6

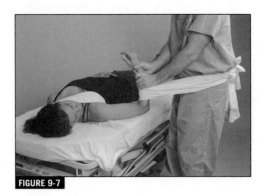

FIGURE 9-7

   d. Place the patient's forearm inside the sheet around your waist so
      that the entire proximal half of the forearm is covered by the sheet
      (Figure 9-7).
4. Apply traction:
   a. Position yourself along the ipsilateral side of the stretcher so that the
      shoulder is slightly abducted.
   b. Lean back slowly and gently to apply traction while providing
      countertraction on the distal half of the forearm with both palms.
      (1) Apply traction over the broadest surface area possible to prevent
          a forearm fracture.
      (2) Be patient; slow, steady traction is necessary to achieve reduction
          (5 to 30 minutes of traction may be required depending on the
          level of sedation).
5. Gently externally rotate the shoulder (Figure 9-8).

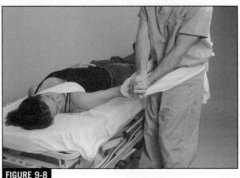

FIGURE 9-8

   a. If reduction not achieved, alternate internal rotation (Figure 9-9) and external rotation.

   b. Vary the degree of abduction if necessary (Figure 9-10).

6. Await a clunk or sudden palpable shift.

7. Gently release traction.

8. Place the arm in a sling (see Chapter 13) in internal rotation or in a gunslinger brace in external rotation.

9. Obtain postreduction radiographs, including an axillary view, before terminating sedation.

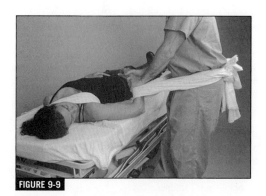

FIGURE 9-9

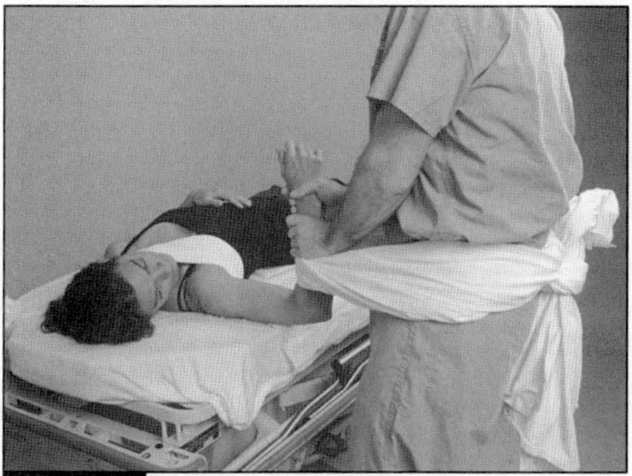

FIGURE 9-10

POSTERIOR GLENOHUMERAL DISLOCATION

Equipment

1. Two bed sheets
2. Stretcher
3. Medications for conscious sedation
4. Sling or gunslinger brace (if available)

Basic Technique

1. Patient positioning:
   a. The patient is supine on a stretcher.
   b. The patient's elbow is bent 90 degrees and the shoulder is internally rotated.
   c. The patient's shoulder is abducted 30 to 60 degrees.
   d. A bed sheet is tied around the patient's trunk and to the opposite side of the stretcher.
   e. A bed sheet is tied around your waist and to the patient's forearm.
2. Landmarks:
   a. Acromion
   b. Humeral head
   c. Coracoid
3. Steps:
   a. Position the patient.
   b. Induce sedation.
   c. Tie the bed sheet to the stretcher.
   d. Tie the bed sheet to yourself.
   e. Lean back to apply traction.
   f. Gently rock the shoulder in slight internal and external rotation.
   g. Once the humeral head is disimpacted, translate the humerus anteriorly.
   h. Gently externally rotate the shoulder.
   i. Await a clunk as the shoulder reduces.
   j. Place the shoulder in a sling or gunslinger brace.
   k. Obtain postreduction films.

Detailed Technique

1. Position the patient supine on the stretcher.
2. Induce conscious sedation.
3. Prepare traction setup:
   a. Make sure guard rails are down on the ipsilateral side and up on the contralateral side.
   b. Slide a rolled bed sheet around the patient's trunk under the ipsilateral shoulder and tie it over the contralateral upper corner of the stretcher for countertraction.
   c. Tie another rolled bed sheet around your waist, leaving about a foot of slack.
   d. Place the patient's forearm inside the sheet around your waist so that the entire proximal half of the forearm is covered by the sheet.

4. Apply traction:
   a. Position yourself along the ipsilateral side of the stretcher so that the shoulder is slightly abducted.
   b. Lean back slowly and gently to apply traction while providing countertraction on the distal half of the forearm with both palms.
      (1) Apply traction over the broadest surface area possible to prevent a forearm fracture.
      (2) Be patient; slow, steady traction is necessary to achieve reduction (5 to 30 minutes of traction may be required depending on the level of sedation).
5. Once the humeral head is disimpacted, translate the humerus anteriorly (Figure 9-11).
6. Gently externally rotate the shoulder.
   a. If reduction is not achieved, alternate internal and external rotation.
   b. Vary the degree of abduction if necessary.
7. Await a clunk or sudden palpable shift.
8. Gently release traction.
9. Place the arm in a sling (see Chapter 13) in internal rotation or in a gunslinger brace in external rotation.
10. Obtain postreduction radiographs, including an axillary view, before terminating sedation.

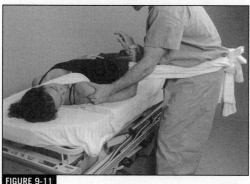

FIGURE 9-11

PROXIMAL HUMERUS FRACTURES

Overview

1. Most proximal humerus fractures require no reduction.
2. Closed reductions of the tuberosities cannot be maintained and should not be attempted (Figure 9-12).
3. Reducing a fracture/dislocation in a closed manner requires a high level of expertise and should only be attempted with caution.
4. Children have a very high remodeling potential at the proximal humerus, and physeal arrest is unlikely.

Indications for Use

Reduction may be indicated for minimally displaced or angulated one- or two-part proximal humerus fractures.

Precautions

Do not attempt heroic measures to reduce proximal humerus fractures.

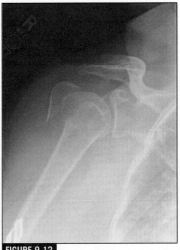

FIGURE 9-12

Pearls

1. Always obtain an axillary view radiograph to rule out a fracture dislocation and to better visualize the humeral head (Figure 9-13).
2. The majority of patients are either older and have low demand because of osteoporosis or are children with high remodeling potential.
3. Use of a sling and swath or a shoulder immobilizer is often definitive treatment.

Improvisation

If no sling and swath or shoulder immobilizer are available, a simple scarf or towel can be used and secured to the body with a loose elastic bandage.

Equipment

1. Sling
2. 6-inch elastic bandages
3. ABD pad with talcum powder (if available)
4. Alternative: shoulder immobilizer

Basic/Detailed Technique

Sling and swath (see Chapter 13).

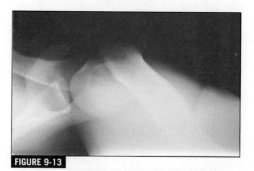

FIGURE 9-13

HUMERAL SHAFT FRACTURES

Overview

1. Most humeral shaft fractures can be treated with closed reduction and splinting/bracing.
2. The radial nerve is closely associated with the humerus and can be injured both from the injury itself and from the reduction attempt.

Indications for Use

Reduction is indicated in all humeral shaft fractures.

Precautions

1. The radial nerve is at risk in this type of fracture and during application of the coaptation splint.
2. A good prereduction and postreduction physical examination is necessary to detail the function of the radial nerve. The radial nerve may be tested by using the following methods:
   a. Thumb extension (Figure 9-14)
   b. Wrist extension (Figure 9-15)
   c. Sensation over the dorsum of the first web space

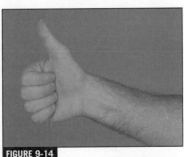

FIGURE 9-14

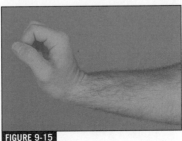

FIGURE 9-15

Pearls

1. Most humeral fractures fall into varus with apex volar deformity (Figure 9-16).
   a. The splint must be applied with a valgus mold to prevent displacement (Figure 9-17).
   b. A pyramidal bump can be placed under the splint to maintain valgus correction (Figures 9-18, 9-19, and 9-20).
2. Distraction is rarely needed and is often counterproductive.

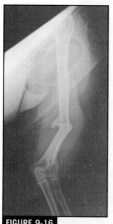

FIGURE 9-16

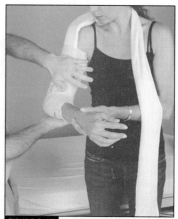

FIGURE 9-17

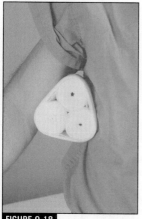

FIGURE 9-18

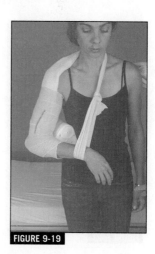

FIGURE 9-19

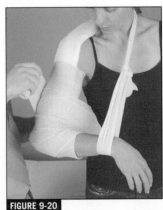

FIGURE 9-20

3. Often it is best to perform the reduction after a coaptation splint is applied but before it sets.
4. Cooperative patients can assist in the reduction by relaxing their shoulder and passively holding their elbow in a flexed position by supporting the injured hand with the uninjured hand.
5. Fractures in the distal third of the diaphysis require immobilization of the elbow in a posterior splint in addition to a coaptation splint.
6. A posterior slab also can be applied because humeral shaft fractures have a tendency to fall into apex anterior angulation (Figures 9-21 and 9-22).

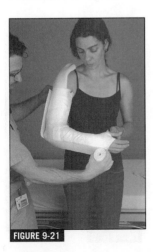

FIGURE 9-21

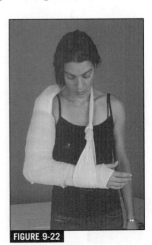

FIGURE 9-22

Improvisation

If supplies are limited, the arm can be sandwiched between two stiff boards or supported by a sling until definitive management can be arranged.

Equipment

1. Stockinette: 4 inches wide and 6 feet long
2. Cast padding: 4 inches wide
3. Plaster: 4 inches wide
4. Elastic or self-adherent bandage: 4 inches wide
5. Tape: 2-inch silk tape (optional)
6. Bucket of tepid water

Basic Technique

1. Patient positioning:
   a. Standing or sitting upright
2. Landmarks:
   a. Acromion
   b. Greater tuberosity of the humerus
   c. Medial and lateral epicondyles
   d. Olecranon process
3. Steps:
   a. Have the patient stand or sit upright.
   b. Apply a coaptation splint.
   c. Perform the reduction maneuver.
   d. Add a bump under the medial elbow if desired.
   e. Bring a stockinette over the contralateral shoulder and tie it to itself to create a sling.

Detailed Technique

1. Apply a coaptation splint (see Chapter 13).
2. Perform a reduction maneuver based on radiographic evidence of displacement. Most fractures require a two-point mold with one hand anterolateral at the fracture site and the other posteromedial at the elbow (Figure 9-23).
3. Bring the excess stockinette material behind the neck and down to and around the wrist and tie it back to itself to create a sling.
4. Create an abduction bump by covering a pyramid of three 4-inch-wide rolls of cast padding in more cast padding.
5. Place the abduction bump between the elbow and the body and secure it to the elbow with elastic or a self-adhesive bandage (see Figure 9-20).
6. A posterior slab may be added to control elbow motion for more distal fractures (see Figure 9-22).
7. Obtain postreduction radiographs.

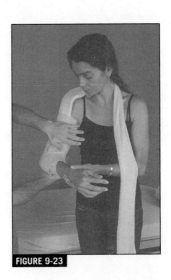

FIGURE 9-23

PERIARTICULAR ELBOW FRACTURES

Overview

1. Most intra-articular elbow fractures require operative treatment.
2. The anterior interosseous nerve (AIN), radial nerve, and ulnar nerves are closely associated with the elbow and are at risk from the injury and the reduction.

Indications for Use

1. Supracondylar humerus fractures
2. Intercondylar humerus fractures (Figure 9-24)
3. Olecranon fractures
4. Radial head/neck fractures

Precautions

Evaluate and document radial nerve, median nerve, ulnar nerve, posterior interosseous nerve (PIN), and AIN function both before and after reduction.

Pearls

1. Reduction techniques should be tailored to the individual fracture pattern.
2. Because distal humeral fractures tend to displace in apex volar angulation, the elbow should be splinted in greater than 90 degrees of flexion.
3. Because proximal ulnar fractures tend to displace in apex dorsal angulation, the elbow should be splinted in less than 90 degrees of flexion in an attempt to reapproximate the fracture fragments.
4. Because radial head/neck fractures tend to displace posteriorly, a reduction maneuver should be attempted before application of a splint.
5. Fractures of the radial head require immobilization of the wrist in a neutral position to prevent pronation and supination.
6. Sometimes it is best to perform the reduction after the splint is applied but before it sets.
7. In the cooperative patient, it is easier to perform the reduction maneuver and apply the splint while the patient is upright.

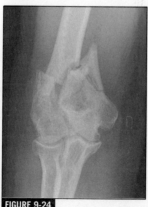

FIGURE 9-24

Improvisation

If supplies are limited, a sling will suffice in an emergency until definitive management can be arranged.

Equipment

Equipment for posterior splint (see Chapter 13)

Basic Technique

1. Patient positioning:
   a. Sitting, supine, or standing
2. Landmarks:
   a. Medial and lateral epicondyles
   b. Olecranon process
   c. Radial head
3. Steps:
   a. Have the patient stand or sit upright or lay supine.
   b. Place the posterior elbow splint with side struts.
   c. Perform a reduction maneuver.
   d. Obtain postreduction films.

Detailed Technique

1. Position the patient standing or sitting upright or supine on a stretcher.
2. Have the patient or an assistant support the arm by holding the wrist if upright.
3. Apply a posterior splint with side struts (see Chapter 13).
4. Perform a reduction maneuver, if warranted, according to the displacement of the fracture (Figure 9-25).
5. Obtain postreduction films.

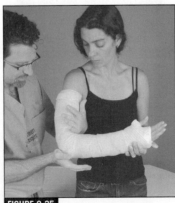

FIGURE 9-25

ELBOW DISLOCATIONS

Overview

1. Elbow dislocations can occur in any direction, but most commonly the ulna dislocates posteriorly (Figure 9-26).
2. The AIN, radial nerve, and ulnar nerve are closely associated with the elbow and are at risk from the injury and the reduction.
3. Most simple elbow dislocations (i.e., those without a fracture) can be treated with a brief period of splinting (1 to 2 weeks) followed by early range of motion.

Indications for Use

1. Elbow dislocations
2. Terrible triad injuries

Precautions

Evaluate and document radial nerve, median nerve, ulnar nerve, PIN, and AIN function both before and after reduction.

Pearls

1. Reduction techniques should be tailored to the direction of the dislocation, with consideration of associated fractures.
2. Terrible triad injuries, which include elbow dislocation, radial head fracture, and coronoid fracture, are extremely unstable injuries, and reduction may not be able to be maintained even in elbow flexion.
3. Terrible triad injuries should be splinted in forearm pronation to tighten the lateral-sided structures.

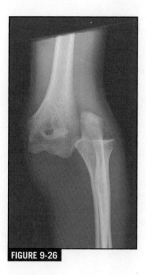

FIGURE 9-26

4. Dislocations with medial epicondyle fractures, which are seen more commonly in children, are associated with ulnar nerve entrapment in the joint. Ulnar nerve dysfunction in this setting is an emergency requiring advanced imaging or exploration.
5. Lateral epicondylar fractures in children are equivalent to lateral ligament ruptures in adults.
6. An unidentified bone fragment anterior to the joint is most commonly a coronoid fracture.
7. In the cooperative patient, it is easier to perform the reduction maneuver and apply the splint while the patient is upright.
8. Immobilization for simple dislocations should be brief and rarely lasts more than 2 weeks.

Improvisation

If supplies are limited, a sling will suffice in an emergency until definitive management can be arranged.

Equipment

Equipment for posterior splint (see Chapter 13)

Basic Technique

1. Patient positioning:
   a. Sitting, supine, or standing
2. Landmarks:
   a. Medial and lateral epicondyles
   b. Olecranon process
   c. Radial head
3. Steps:
   a. Have the patient stand or sit upright or lay supine.
   b. Prepare the splint.
   c. Perform a reduction maneuver.
   d. Place a posterior elbow splint with side bars.
   e. Obtain postreduction films.

Detailed Technique

1. Position the patient standing or sitting upright if a hematoma block is to be used for anesthesia (in a cooperative patient).
2. Position the patient supine on a stretcher with the ipsilateral shoulder off the stretcher if conscious sedation is to be used.
3. Prepare splinting material (see Chapter 13).
4. Stand at the side of the bed, facing the elbow.
5. If any medial/lateral translation is present, stabilize the distal humerus with one hand while grasping the proximal forearm with the other hand (Figure 9-27).
6. While applying gentle traction, translate the forearm on the humerus.
7. Feel the epicondyles and the olecranon to ensure that the olecranon is between the two epicondyles.

8. Place one hand anterior on the distal humerus and the other hand grasping the wrist (**Figure 9-28**).
9. With the elbow held in extension, pull hard manual traction across the elbow.
10. While pushing down on the distal humerus, begin flexing the elbow while maintaining traction (**Figure 9-29**).
11. A clunk may be felt when the joint is reduced, but a clunk does not always occur.
12. If the elbow can be fully flexed with no crepitus, it is most likely reduced (**Figure 9-30**).
13. Have an assistant hold the elbow in at least 90 degrees of flexion and forearm pronation.
14. Apply a posterior splint (see Chapter 13).
15. Obtain postreduction films.

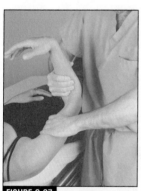

FIGURE 9-27

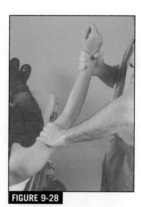

FIGURE 9-28

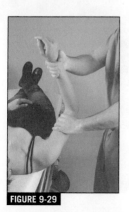

FIGURE 9-29

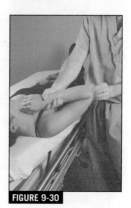

FIGURE 9-30

RADIAL HEAD DISLOCATION

Overview

1. Radial head dislocations can occur posteriorly, laterally, and anteriorly.
2. The PIN is at risk from the injury and the reduction.
3. Most radial heads can be reduced in a closed manner without the need for surgical intervention.
4. Closed reduction failure usually results from either the radial head buttonholing through the capsule or an ulnar fracture or plastic deformation limiting reduction.

Indications for Use

1. Radial head dislocation without associated fractures
2. "Nursemaid's elbow"

Precautions

1. Evaluate and document radial nerve, median nerve, ulnar nerve, PIN, and AIN function both before and after reduction.
2. Do not try to reduce a chronically dislocated radial head; a careful history, lack of pain, and radiographs demonstrating a convex radial head articulation will provide evidence of a long-standing dislocation.

Pearls

1. Make sure that the ulna is not fractured and that a Monteggia injury has not occurred.
2. Beware of the plastically deformed ulna:
   a. This Monteggia variant will not allow closed reduction of the radial head without correction of the ulnar alignment (Figure 9-31).

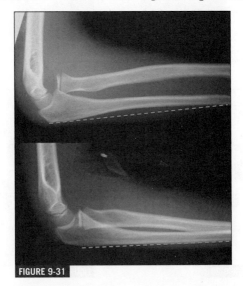

FIGURE 9-31

  b. Note that the ulna does not form a straight line along the posterior
     border (as shown by the dotted lines in Figure 9-31).
3. Evaluate postreduction films for evidence of a radial head and/or
   coronoid fracture to rule out a terrible triad injury.

Improvisation

No harm can come from trying other maneuvers in the search for a
reduction.

Equipment

Equipment for a posterior splint (see Chapter 13)

Basic Technique

1. Patient positioning:
   a. Sitting, supine, or standing
2. Landmarks:
   a. Medial and lateral epicondyles
   b. Olecranon process
   c. Radial head
3. Steps:
   a. Have the patient stand or sit upright or lay supine.
   b. Prepare a splint.
   c. Perform a reduction maneuver.
   d. Place a posterior elbow splint with side bars.
   e. Obtain postreduction films.

Detailed Technique

1. Position the patient standing or sitting upright if a hematoma block is to
   be used for anesthesia (in a cooperative patient).
2. Position the patient supine on a stretcher with the ipsilateral shoulder off
   the stretcher if conscious sedation is to be used.
3. Have the patient or an assistant support the arm by holding the wrist
   upright.
4. Prepare splinting materials (see Chapter 13).
5. Stand at the side of the bed, facing the elbow.

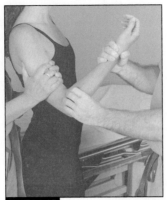

FIGURE 9-32

6. Anterior dislocation:
   a. While an assistant stabilizes the arm, flex the arm past 90 degrees to relax the biceps, then supinate the forearm while applying direct, posteriorly directed pressure to the radial head and pulling traction at the wrist (Figure 9-32).
7. Posterior dislocation:
   a. While an assistant stabilizes the arm, place the biceps on tension by extending the elbow and pronating the forearm.
   b. Apply traction and a slight varus movement while placing an anteriorly directed force directly on the radial head (Figure 9-33).

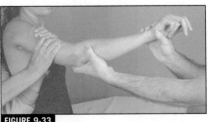

FIGURE 9-33

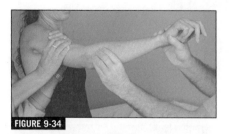

FIGURE 9-34

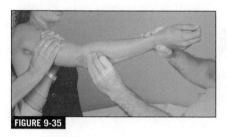

FIGURE 9-35

8. Lateral dislocation:
   a. While an assistant stabilizes the arm, extend the elbow and pronate (Figure 9-34) or supinate (Figure 9-35) the forearm depending on whether a posterior or anterior movement is desired.
   b. Apply traction and a slight varus movement while placing a medially directed force directly on the radial head.
9. A clunk may be felt when the joint is reduced, but not always.
10. Maintain the elbow in the forearm rotation required for reduction.
11. Apply a posterior splint with side struts if desired (see Chapter 13).
12. Obtain postreduction radiographs.

Chapter 10
Forearm, Wrist, and Hand Reduction

FOREARM FRACTURES

Overview

1. Fractures of both bones of the forearm (Figure 10-1) should be reduced anatomically (except in children younger than 12 years) to preserve forearm rotation.
   a. Only accept as much deformity as can remodel in 1 year.
   b. In children younger than 8 years, bayonet apposition and 20 degrees of angulation is acceptable.
   c. In children older than approximately 8 years, length should be restored and angulation of 10 degrees is acceptable.
2. A Monteggia fracture is a combination of a radial head dislocation and a fracture of the ulna. The vast majority of Monteggia fractures should be treated surgically.
   a. Anatomic reduction of the ulnar fracture often results in spontaneous reduction of the radiocapitellar dislocation.
   b. In children, a greenstick fracture of the ulna may occur or the ulna may plastically deform, and the radial head dislocation is often missed (Figure 10-2).

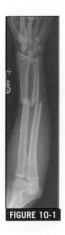

FIGURE 10-1

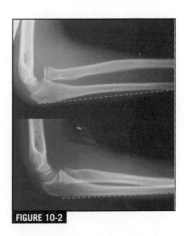

FIGURE 10-2

   c. The direction of radial head displacement and ulnar fracture
      angulation varies and dictates the reduction maneuvers.
3. A Galeazzi fracture is a combination of a radial fracture and a distal
   radioulnar joint dislocation.
   a. The vast majority of Galeazzi fractures should be treated surgically.
   b. Anatomic reduction of the radial fracture often results in spontaneous
      reduction of the distal radioulnar joint dislocation.
4. Nightstick fractures of the diaphyseal ulna can accommodate 10
   degrees of angulation and 50% translation.

Indications for Use

1. Ulnar shaft fractures with or without radial head dislocation
2. Radial shaft fractures with or without distal radioulnar joint dislocation
3. Fractures of both bones of the forearm

Precautions

1. Even if an anatomic reduction is achieved, follow-up should occur within
   a week of the injury.
2. Do not use an intravenous (IV) stand that is attached to the ceiling
   unless it is specifically designed to handle large weights.
3. Ensure that the finger trap is secure! Sudden and unanticipated
   release of traction can result in injury to both the patient and the
   physician.

Pearls

1. Patient positioning is key to obtaining appropriate traction. Strict
   positioning of the shoulder to 90 degrees and flexion of the elbow to 90
   degrees allows perfectly longitudinal traction to be applied through the
   fracture site.
2. Be patient! Allow 5 to 10 minutes for traction to result in disimpaction of
   the fracture.
3. Forewarn patients that their index and long fingers may hurt more than
   their forearms by virtue of the finger trap.
   a. Also inform patients that their fingers will likely turn blue but that this
      symptom is normal, expected, and will resolve shortly after the finger
      traps are removed.
   b. Performing a digital block of the index and long fingers before traction
      may be considered in certain patients.
4. To "release traction" while performing the reduction maneuver, it is
   often easier to simply grasp the hand and allow slack in the fingertrap or
   traction loop.

Improvisation

1. Reduction of a forearm fracture requires tailoring the technique to each fracture type.
2. If supplies are limited, taping the forearm to a stiff board will suffice until definitive management can be arranged.
3. Alternative reduction methods can be attempted if no traction is available.
   a. Grasp the proximal forearm and the distal forearm with the thumb of the proximal hand just proximal to the fracture site (Figure 10-3).
   b. Pull traction while using your thumb to key in the fracture by pushing on the proximal fragment at the fracture apex (Figure 10-4).

Equipment

1. Stockinette: 3 inches wide, 4 feet long
2. Rolled gauze: 2 inches wide
3. IV pole
4. Weights: 10 to 15 lb
5. ABD pad (optional)

Basic Technique

1. Patient positioning:
   a. Supine on stretcher
   b. Shoulder to 90 degrees and flexion of elbow to 90 degrees
2. Landmarks:
   a. Ulnar head
   b. Radial head
   c. Radial styloid
   d. Subcutaneous border of ulna

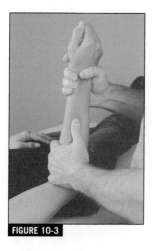

FIGURE 10-3

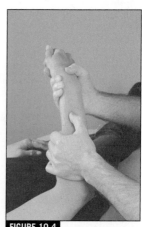

FIGURE 10-4

3. Steps:
   a. Position the patient.
   b. Prepare finger traps.
   c. Set traction, if necessary.
   d. Obtain traction views, if desired.
   e. If a long arm cast will be applied afterward, place cast padding on the elbow and proximal surface before applying traction.
   f. Perform a reduction maneuver.
   g. Apply a cast or splint.
   h. Remove traction.
   i. Obtain elbow, forearm, and wrist films.

Detailed Technique

1. Position the patient:
   a. The patient should be supine on the stretcher with his or her shoulder girdle entirely off the side.
   b. If a long arm cast will be applied afterward, place a stockinette (see Chapter 13).
2. Begin sedation.
3. Prepare finger traps:
   a. Attach a rolled gauze finger trap (Chapter 8) to the index and long fingers using a double-ring construct (Figure 10-5).
   b. Abduct the shoulder to 90 degrees and flex the elbow to 90 degrees to create a 90-90 position.
   c. Secure the other end of the traction to the IV pole.
4. Set traction, if necessary (Figure 10-6).
   a. Cut a 2-foot length of stockinette.

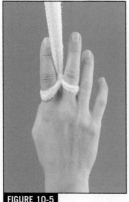

FIGURE 10-5

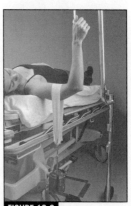

FIGURE 10-6

   b. Place an ABD inside the stockinette for padding (optional).

   c. Cut small holes in each end of the stockinette.

   d. Drape the stockinette around the forearm.

   e. Hang the traction weights.

   f. Allow traction to hang for at least 5 minutes (less than 1 hour is recommended).

5. Obtain traction views (optional). Portable anteroposterior (AP) and lateral radiographs of the forearm, wrist, and elbow can be obtained in traction to evaluate the reduction.

6. Perform a reduction maneuver (Figures 10-7 and 10-8).

   a. The direction in which forces are applied depends on the type of fracture.

   b. Bring the distal fragment to the proximal fragment.

   c. Correct forearm rotation to match proximal fragments, generally as described below:

     (1) Proximal fractures of both bones of the forearm: mild supination

     (2) Midshaft fractures of both bones of the forearm: neutral

     (3) Distal fractures of both bones of the forearm: slight pronation

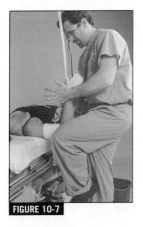

FIGURE 10-7

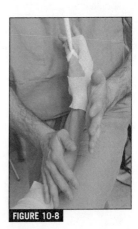

FIGURE 10-8

7. Apply a splint (see Chapter 13) or a cast (see Chapter 13) while maintaining traction.
   a. Prepare an interosseous mold (Figure 10-9).
   b. Flatten the ulnar border of the cast/splint with your shin (Figure 10-10) or a flat surface (Figure 10-11).
8. Obtain postreduction AP and lateral films of the elbow, forearm, and wrist.

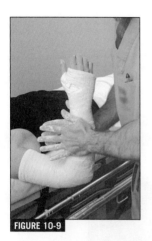

FIGURE 10-9

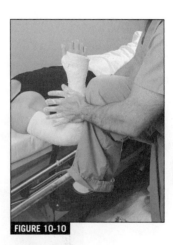

FIGURE 10-10

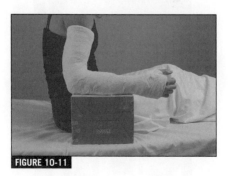

FIGURE 10-11

DISTAL RADIUS FRACTURE REDUCTION

Overview

1. Many distal radius fractures, particularly in children, can be treated with closed reduction and casting (Figure 10-12).
2. The principle of the distal radius fracture reduction method is to:
   a. Disimpact the fracture by using hanging traction
   b. Manually reduce the distal fragment
3. This procedure can be performed by a single individual when an IV pole and traction weights are used.

Indications for Use

1. Displaced distal radius fractures
2. Carpal fractures

Precautions

1. Do not use an IV stand attached to the ceiling unless it is specifically designed to handle large weights.
2. Ensure that the finger trap is secure! A sudden and unanticipated release of traction can result in injury to both the patient and the physician.

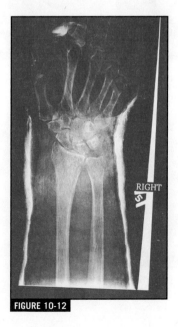

FIGURE 10-12

Pearls

1. Patient positioning is key to obtaining appropriate traction. Strict positioning of the shoulder to 90 degrees and flexion of the elbow to 90 degrees allows perfectly longitudinal traction to be applied through the fracture site.
2. Be patient! Allow 5 to 10 minutes for traction to result in disimpaction of the fracture.
3. Forewarn patients that their thumb may hurt more than their wrist by virtue of the finger trap.
   a. Also inform patients that their thumb will likely turn blue but that this symptom is normal, expected, and will resolve shortly after the finger traps are removed.
   b. Performing a digital block of the thumb before traction may be considered in certain patients.
4. To "release traction" while performing the reduction maneuver, it is often easiest to simply grasp the forearm and allow slack on the finger trap or traction loop.

Improvisation

1. Alternative reduction methods can be attempted if traction is not available or is ineffective.
   a. Alternative 1: Use your thenar eminences to "contour" the forearm and apply traction if minimal displacement is present (Figure 10-13).
   b. Alternative 2: If the fracture is bayoneted:
      (1) Grasp the forearm and the palm with the thumb of the proximal hand just proximal to the fracture site (Figure 10-14).

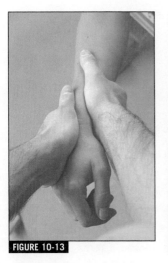

FIGURE 10-13

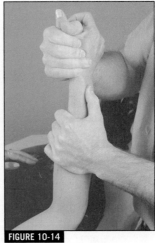

FIGURE 10-14

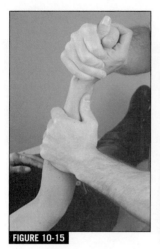

FIGURE 10-15

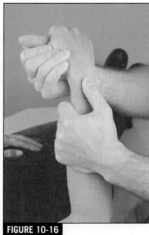

FIGURE 10-16

(2) Recreate the injury by extending the fracture, using your thumb as the fulcrum (Figure 10-15).

(3) Once the fragments unlock, pull as much manual traction as possible and flex the wrist while advancing your thumb distalward and applying a volarly directed force to the distal fracture fragment (Figure 10-16).

2. If a weight pole is not available, see Chapter 12.

Equipment

1. Stockinette: 3 inches wide, 4 feet long
2. Rolled gauze: 2 inches wide
3. IV pole
4. Weights: 10 to 15 lb
5. ABD (optional)

Basic Technique

1. Patient positioning:
   a. Supine on stretcher
   b. Shoulder to 90 degrees and flexion of elbow to 90 degrees
2. Landmarks:
   a. Lister's tubercle (often obscured by swelling)
   b. Radial styloid
3. Steps:
   a. Position the patient.
   b. Prepare finger traps.
   c. Set traction, if necessary.
   d. Obtain traction films, if desired.
   e. If a long arm cast will be applied afterward, apply cast padding.

  f. Perform a reduction maneuver.
  g. Holding your thumb on the fracture site, use your knee to help maintain the wrist in a flexed posture while traction is reapplied.

Detailed Technique

1. Position the patient:
   a. The patient should be supine on the stretcher with the shoulder girdle entirely off the side.
   b. If a long arm cast will be applied afterward, place a stockinette (see Chapter 13).
2. Prepare finger trap:
   a. Attach a rolled gauze fingertrap (see Chapter 8) to the thumb using a single-ring construct (Figure 10-17).
   b. Abduct the shoulder to 90 degrees and flex the elbow to 90 degrees to create a 90-90 position.
   c. Secure the other end of the rolled gauze to the IV pole.
   d. Alternatively, commercially available finger traps may be used. However, we have found that commercial finger traps are liable to loosening during traction application.
3. Set traction, if necessary:
   a. Cut a 2-foot length of stockinette.
   b. Place an ABD inside the stockinette for padding (optional).
   c. Cut small holes in each end of the stockinette.
   d. Drape the stockinette around the forearm.
   e. Hang the traction weights.
   f. Allow the traction weights to hang for at least 5 minutes.

10

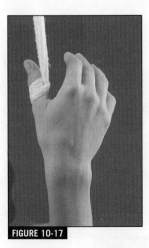

FIGURE 10-17

4. Obtain traction films (optional). Portable AP and lateral radiographs of the distal radius should be obtained while the patient is in traction.
5. Perform a reduction maneuver.
   a. The direction in which forces are applied depends on the type of distal radius fracture.
      (1) Because the majority of distal radius fractures are displaced dorsally, the description below applies to a dorsally displaced distal radius fracture.
      (2) For volarly displaced fractures, reverse the direction.
   b. Grasp the hand, as if arm wrestling, using your right hand.
   c. With your left hand, grasp the proximal radius with your thumb on the fracture site dorsally and your fingers curled around the radius proximal to the fracture (see Figure 10-14).
   d. Recreate the mechanism by hyperextending the wrist (see Figure 10-15).
   e. Release the hanging traction temporarily. Pull up with your right hand.
   f. Begin to flex the wrist.
   g. Shift your thumb slightly distally so it is over the distal fragment.
   h. Using your left thumb, push the fragment volarward and use your fingers to pull dorsalward (see Figure 10-16).
6. Holding your thumb on the fracture site, use your knee to help maintain the wrist in a flexed posture while traction is reapplied. This technique maintains the reduction.
7. Apply a splint or cast (see Chapter 13).
8. Place a three-point mold on the splint, ensuring that the wrist is in slight flexion and moderate ulnar deviation and that the carpals are translated volarly (Figure 10-18).

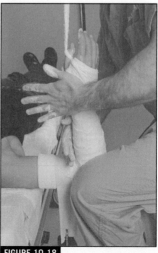

FIGURE 10-18

INTERCARPAL DISLOCATION

Overview

Intercarpal dislocations are illustrated in **Figures 10-19 and 10-20**.

1. Intercarpal dislocations are often missed in the emergency setting.
2. All intercarpal dislocations require urgent operative fixation.
3. Reducing the dislocation by closed means is extremely difficult.
4. Use of general anesthesia or conscious sedation often is helpful in obtaining the reduction.

Indications for Use

1. Lesser arc injuries (perilunate or lunate dislocations)
2. Greater arc injuries (perilunate or lunate dislocations with associated carpal fractures)

Precautions

1. Do not use an IV stand attached to the ceiling unless it is specifically designed to handle large weights.
2. Ensure that the finger trap is secure! Sudden and unanticipated release of traction can result in injury to both the patient and the physician.

Pearls

1. Patient positioning is key to obtaining appropriate traction. Strict positioning of the shoulder to 90 degrees and flexion of elbow to 90 degrees allows perfectly longitudinal traction to be applied through the fracture site.
2. Be patient! Allow at least 20 minutes for traction to result in exhaustion of countering muscles.
3. Forewarn patients that their fingers may hurt more than their wrist by virtue of the finger trap.
4. Also inform patients that their fingers will likely turn blue but that this symptom is normal, expected, and will resolve shortly after the finger traps are removed.

10

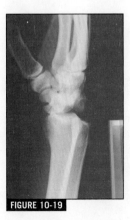

FIGURE 10-19

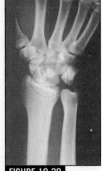

FIGURE 10-20

5. To "release traction" while performing the reduction maneuver, it is often easiest to simply grasp the forearm and allow slack in the rolled gauze.

Improvisation

If a weight pole is not available, see Chapter 8.

Equipment

1. Stockinette: 3 inches wide, 4 feet long
2. Rolled gauze: 2 inches wide
3. IV pole
4. Weights: 10 to 15 lb
5. ABD pad (optional)

Basic Technique

1. Patient positioning:
   a. Supine on stretcher
   b. Shoulder to 90 degrees and flexion of elbow to 90 degrees
2. Landmarks:
   a. Lister's tubercle (often obscured by swelling)
   b. Radial styloid
   c. Scaphoid tubercle
3. Steps:
   a. Position the patient.
   b. Prepare finger traps.
   c. Set traction.
   d. Perform a reduction maneuver.
   e. Obtain postreduction films while the patient is in traction if possible.
   f. Apply cast padding.
   g. Place a sugar-tong splint.
   h. Release traction.
   i. Obtain postreduction films.

Detailed Technique

1. Position the patient supine on the stretcher with his or her shoulder girdle entirely off the side.
2. Prepare finger trap:
   a. Attach the rolled gauze to the index and long fingers using a double-ring construct.
      (1) Make a loop of gauze.
      (2) Place the loop around the thumb.
      (3) While holding one side of the gauze taut, place your other hand into the loop.
      (4) Spread your fingers and pull upward.
      (5) Hook one ring around each finger.
      (6) Pull the free end taut.

   b. Abduct the shoulder to 90 degrees and flex the elbow to 90 degrees to create a 90-90 position.

   c. Secure the other end of the gauze to the IV pole.

   d. Alternatively, commercially available Chinese finger traps may be used. However, we have found that these finger traps are liable to loosen during application of traction.

3. Set traction, if necessary.

   a. Cut a 2-foot length of stockinette.

   b. Place an ABD inside the stockinette for padding (optional).

   c. Cut small holes in each end of the stockinette.

   d. Drape the stockinette around the forearm.

   e. Hang the traction weights.

   f. Allow the traction weights to hang for at least 20 minutes.

4. Perform a reduction maneuver.

   a. Have an assistant stabilize the arm by placing both hands over the brachium.

   b. Grasp the patient's hand with one hand to apply traction.

   c. With the other hand, grasp the distal forearm so that your thumb points toward the traction, coming to rest at the distal wrist crease.

   d. Extend the wrist while applying pressure on the lunate with your thumb (Figure 10-21).

   e. While applying maximal manual traction and maintaining pressure on the lunate with your thumb, bring the wrist back to neutral or slight flexion (Figure 10-22).

10

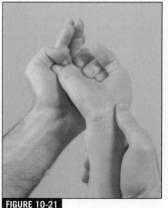

FIGURE 10-21

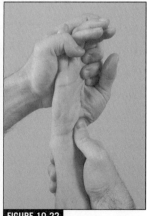

FIGURE 10-22

5. Obtain postreduction views while the patient is in traction if possible. Portable AP and lateral radiographs of the carpals can be obtained while the patient is in traction.
6. Apply a sugar-tong splint (see Chapter 13) while maintaining the wrist in slight flexion and ulnar deviation.
7. Obtain postreduction films.

BOXER'S FRACTURE

Overview

Boxer's fracture is illustrated in **Figure 10-23**.

1. Fractures of the fifth metacarpal neck are easy to reduce, but maintaining the reduction with closed means is unlikely.
2. Angulation of up to 45 degrees is usually well tolerated.
3. An ulnar nerve block provides complete pain relief of the fifth metacarpal.

Indications for Use

1. Fourth or fifth metacarpal shaft fractures
2. Fourth or fifth metacarpal neck fractures

Precautions

The molding required to hold a reduction can lead to pressure necrosis of the dorsal skin and extensor tendons.

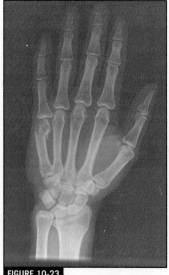

FIGURE 10-23

Pearls

1. Ensure that rotational alignment is perfect by checking to be certain that no scissoring of the digits occurs when the patient makes a fist.
2. Augment analgesia with a hematoma block when reducing the fourth metacarpal.
3. Immobilizing the proximal interphalangeal (PIP) joints is not necessary if the proximal phalanx is not fractured.

Improvisation

The fracture is usually minimally painful and can await definitive management if supplies are not available.

Equipment

1. Ulnar gutter cast (see Chapter 13)
2. Ulnar gutter splint (see Chapter 13)

Basic Technique

1. Patient positioning:
   a. Supine on stretcher, standing, or sitting upright
2. Landmarks:
   a. Fifth and fourth metacarpal heads
   b. Fifth and fourth metacarpal shafts
   c. Fifth and fourth digit proximal phalanges
3. Steps:
   a. Position the patient.
   b. Perform an ulnar nerve block.
   c. Perform a reduction maneuver.
   d. Apply cast padding.
   e. Place an ulnar gutter splint or cast.
   f. Obtain postreduction films.

Detailed Technique

1. Position the patient so the forearm is vertical.
2. Perform a field block, nerve block, or hematoma block. An ulnar nerve block is reliable for fifth metacarpal fractures, but fourth metacarpal fractures may need a supplemental field or hematoma block.

3. Perform a reduction maneuver (Figure 10-24).
   a. With one hand, stabilize the patient's hand by pinching the metacarpal between your thumb and index fingers.
   b. With your other hand, curl the patient's affected finger and apply a dorsally directed force on the proximal phalanx.
4. Place an ulnar gutter splint or cast (see Chapter 13).
5. Place a mold on the splint/cast (Figure 10-25).
   a. Place your left thumb just proximal to or at the apex of the fracture.
   b. Grasp all the fingers in your right palm and apply a dorsally directed force while maintaining the metacarpophalangeal (MP) joints flexed and the interphalangeal (IP) joints in an extended position.
6. Obtain postreduction films.

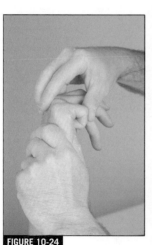

FIGURE 10-24

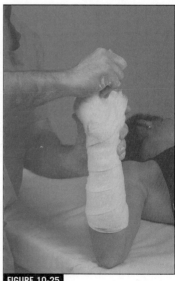

FIGURE 10-25

DIGITAL DISLOCATIONS

Overview

1. Digital dislocations can occur from either axial load or hyperextension/ hyperflexion.
2. Once reduced, most digital dislocations are stable at rest but should be protected from subsequent injury with a short course of splinting.
3. Radiographs often will demonstrate a concomitant intra-articular fracture.
   a. A small fleck of bone off the dorsal or volar aspect of a joint represents a ligament or tendon avulsion and does not alter management.
   b. A true fracture/dislocation involving more than 20% of the articular surface (Figure 10-26) may be inherently unstable and should prompt an urgent visit to a hand surgeon.

Indications for Use

1. Thumb MP dislocations
2. Thumb IP dislocations
3. Finger MP dislocations
4. Finger PIP dislocations
5. Finger distal IP dislocations

Precautions

Hyperextension of a digit in a dorsal splint can lead to pressure necrosis of the dorsal skin and extensor tendons.

10

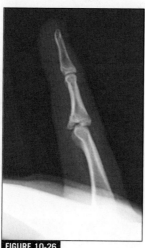

FIGURE 10-26

Pearls

1. A good block is essential to permit application of sufficient traction and force to reduce the dislocations.
2. In-line traction is typically sufficient to reduce most dislocations (Figure 10-27).

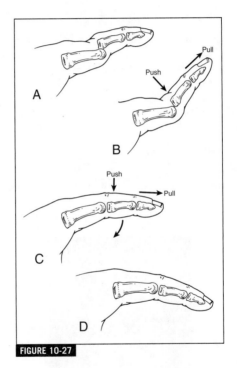

FIGURE 10-27

3. Recreating the mechanism of injury while applying traction can be helpful (Figure 10-28).

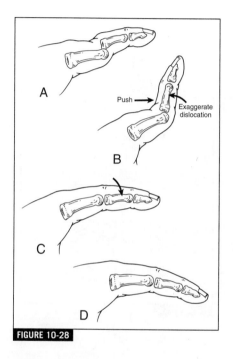

FIGURE 10-28

4. For thumb MP dislocations, placing the wrist and IP joint in flexion releases tension on the flexor pollicis longus and aids in the reduction (Figure 10-29).

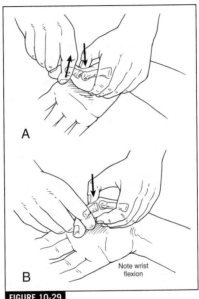

FIGURE 10-29

5. If a reduction cannot be achieved, consider the possibility that soft tissue (e.g., volar plate or tendons) is interposed or that the bone is buttonholed between two tendons (Figure 10-30).
6. If the fracture/dislocation or dislocation reduces but then redisplaces even in the splint, it is inherently unstable and requires urgent attention by a hand surgeon.

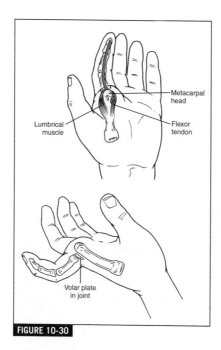

FIGURE 10-30

Improvisation

If at first you don't succeed, try something else.

Equipment

1. Aluminum padded splint
2. ½-inch-wide silk tape

Basic Technique

1. Patient positioning:
   a. Supine on stretcher, standing, or sitting upright
2. Landmarks:
   a. Digital condyles
   b. Metacarpal head
3. Steps:
   a. Position the patient.
   b. Perform a nerve block.
   c. Precut strips of tape to 3 inches in length.
   d. Prepare an aluminum foam splint.
   e. Perform a reduction maneuver.
   f. Apply the aluminum splint.
   g. Secure the splint in place with tape.
   h. Obtain postreduction films.

Detailed Technique

1. Position the patient so that you have direct access to his or her fingers.
2. Perform a nerve block.
   a. An ulnar nerve block is reliable for the small finger.
   b. Median and radial nerve blocks at the wrist are necessary for thumb dislocations.
   c. Digital blocks are sufficient for finger dislocations.
   d. Wait 10 to 15 minutes for the nerve block to take effect.

3. Precut strips of ½-inch silk tape into 3-inch lengths.
4. Measure the aluminum foam splint and cut it to size (Figure 10-31). Only the involved joint should be splinted.
5. Trim away excess foam (Figure 10-32).

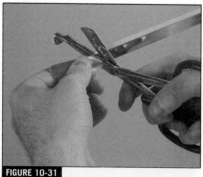

FIGURE 10-31

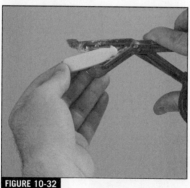

FIGURE 10-32

6. Contour the splint with an appropriate bend.
   a. Dorsal dislocations (distal bone dislocates dorsally) can be splinted in flexion (Figure 10-33) or extension block splints (Figure 10-34).
   b. Volar dislocations (distal bone dislocates volarly) should be splinted in extension (Figure 10-35).

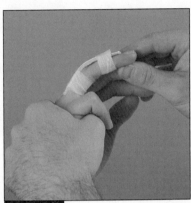

FIGURE 10-33

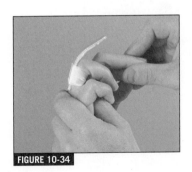

FIGURE 10-34

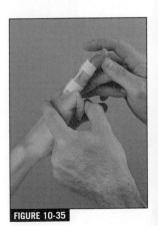

FIGURE 10-35

7. Perform reduction maneuver:
   a. Finger MP joints:
      (1) With one hand, stabilize the patient's hand.
      (2) Pinch the finger with your other hand and apply traction (Figure 10-36).
      (3) Exaggerate the deformity if necessary.
   b. Thumb MP joints:
      (1) With one hand, stabilize the patient's hand.
      (2) Pinch the thumb with your other hand and apply traction (Figure 10-37).
      (3) Exaggerate the deformity if necessary.
      (4) Flexion of the wrist and IP joint can facilitate reduction (see Figure 10-29).

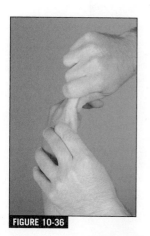

FIGURE 10-36

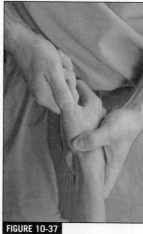

FIGURE 10-37

   c. Finger IP joints:
     (1) With one hand, stabilize the patient's hand.
     (2) Pinch the finger with your other hand and apply traction (Figure 10-38).
     (3) Exaggerate the deformity if necessary.
   d. Thumb IP joint:
     (1) With one hand, stabilize the patient's hand.
     (2) Pinch the finger with your other hand and apply traction.
     (3) Exaggerate the deformity if necessary.
8. Place a padded aluminum splint for IP joint dislocations.
   a. Hold the splint in place while applying circumferential tape.
   b. Securing the distal end of the splint first is easiest (Figure 10-39).
9. Obtain postreduction films.

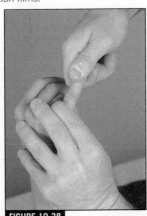

FIGURE 10-38

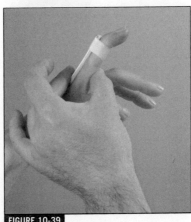

FIGURE 10-39

Chapter 11
Pelvis and Lower Extremity Reduction

PELVIS REDUCTION

Overview

1. Application of a pelvic binder is a key step in the initial management of an unstable pelvic fracture.
2. Commercial pelvic binders are available, or a simple bed sheet may be used as a pelvic binder.
3. Venous bleeding is the most common cause of hemorrhage in a patient with hemodynamic instability and an unstable pelvic fracture.
4. By applying a binder, stability is provided to the fracture, allowing tamponade and organization of the hematoma.

Indications for Use

Unstable "open book" pelvic injury (Tile B injury or anterior-posterior compression [APC] II or III injuries)
1. Note that placement of a pelvic binder is not contraindicated in a patient with a lateral compression–type injury.
2. The benefit of using a pelvic binder for a lateral compression–type injury is not likely to be as great as for an open book pelvic injury.

Precautions

1. Close coordination with the trauma team and trauma anesthesiologist is mandatory.
2. Perform a careful physical examination before applying a binder. Determine if the fracture is open or closed.
3. Correct placement of a pelvic binder is vital for it to function properly.
   a. The binder should be centered around the greater trochanters.
   b. The binder should *not* be centered at the patient's waist.

Pearls

1. Although commercial binders are easier to apply than a bed sheet, not all emergency departments are equipped with commercial binders, so it is important to know how to use both a commercial binder and a bed sheet.
2. Place a towel over the perineal area to protect the structures therein.
3. After a commercial binder or a bed sheet is placed, postreduction radiographs are mandatory.
4. If the sheet will be used for more than emergent stabilization, use two to four towel clips rather than tying the sheet to prevent loosening and pressure necrosis.

Equipment

1. Two people are required to reduce the pelvis and apply a binder appropriately (not shown).
2. Commercial pelvic binder (Figure 11-1) or a bed sheet
3. Towel clamps, Kelly forceps, or other large clamps

Basic Technique

1. Patient positioning:
   a. Supine on stretcher
2. Landmarks:
   a. Greater trochanters
   b. Anterior superior iliac spines (ASIS)
3. Steps:
   a. Position the patient.
   b. Palpate landmarks.
   c. Roll the patient.
   d. Reduce the pelvis.
   e. Place the commercial binder or bed sheet.

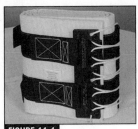

FIGURE 11-1

Detailed Technique

1. Position the patient.
2. Palpate landmarks; feel both greater trochanters and ASIS (Figure 11-2).
3. Roll the patient. A standard trauma log-roll technique should be used to place the commercial binder or bed sheet under the patient (Figure 11-3), with additional people at the legs and the head.
4. If a bed sheet is being used, place it as widely as possible over the greater trochanter and ASIS.
   a. Reduce the pelvis by applying an inward force.
   b. Use towel clips if available. If not, tie a very tight knot around the pelvis and add a second square knot (Figure 11-4).

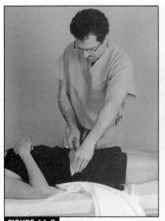

FIGURE 11-2

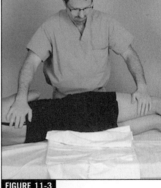

FIGURE 11-3

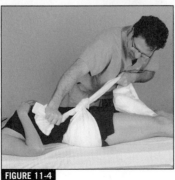

FIGURE 11-4

5. Procedure for placing a commercial binder:
   a. Wrap the binder around the patient (Figure 11-5).
   b. Ensure correct placement. The binder must be centered on the greater trochanters.
   c. Trim any excess (Figure 11-6).
   d. Reduce the pelvis by applying an inward force.
   e. Pull the cords to tighten the binder (Figure 11-7).

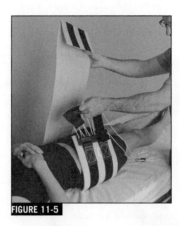

FIGURE 11-5

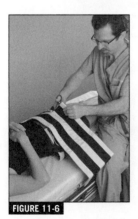

FIGURE 11-6

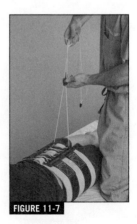

FIGURE 11-7

HIP REDUCTION

Overview

1. Numerous maneuvers have been described for reduction of dislocated hips.
2. All maneuvers basically function to recreate the deforming force.
   a. Posterior dislocations (Figure 11-8): flexion, adduction, and internal rotation
   b. Anterior dislocations: abduction and external rotation in extension
3. The incidence of dislocated hips is much higher in patients with hip arthroplasty compared with patients who do not have hip arthroplasty.
4. The vast majority of hip dislocations are directed posteriorly.
5. Relocation of hips can be difficult because of the significant muscular and ligamentous impediments inherent to the joint.
6. In patients with traumatic dislocations, relocation is easier because of the associated posterior wall acetabular fracture.

Indications for Use

Posterior hip dislocation using the modified Bigelow technique

Precautions

An assistant is required for the modified Bigelow to apply countertraction.

Pearls

Conscious sedation is virtually mandatory in most patients. The typical exception to this rule is a patient with a total hip arthroplasty whose hip becomes dislocated on a chronic basis.

Equipment

Bed sheet

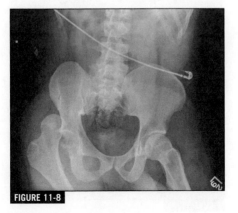

FIGURE 11-8

Basic Technique

1. Patient positioning:
   a. Supine on stretcher
2. Landmarks:
   a. Anterior superior iliac spine
   b. Greater trochanters
3. Steps:
   a. Obtain conscious sedation.
   b. Position the patient.
   c. Perform a reduction maneuver.
   d. Apply an abduction pillow.

Detailed Technique

1. Obtain conscious sedation.
2. Position the patient. The patient should be completely supine.
3. Tie a bed sheet loosely around your waist (Figure 11-9).
4. Perform a reduction maneuver:
   a. The surgeon mounts the stretcher and straddles the affected extremity between his or her legs (Figure 11-10).

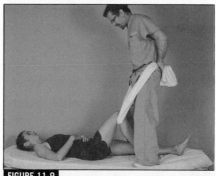
FIGURE 11-9

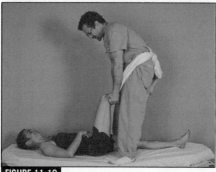
FIGURE 11-10

b. The patient's knee is flexed to 90 degrees, and the hip is also flexed to 90 degrees.
c. The surgeon's arms are locked together under the knee.
d. An assistant applies countertraction via the ASIS (Figure 11-11).
e. The surgeon applies an upwardly directed force.
f. The hip is then adducted.
g. The hip is then internally rotated (Figure 11-12).
h. Once the hip is reduced in this position:
  (1) Maintain traction and externally rotate and abduct the hip.
  (2) Bring the hip into extension.
  (3) Apply an abduction pillow if appropriate.

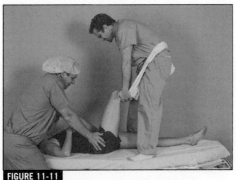

FIGURE 11-11

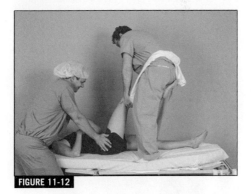

FIGURE 11-12

KNEE REDUCTION

Overview

1. Dislocation of the knee is associated with a high incidence of associated vascular and nerve injuries. The popliteal artery and peroneal nerve are most commonly injured.
2. The overall management of a patient with a knee dislocation is of paramount importance compared with the actual reduction maneuver.
   a. Many knee dislocations can be reduced easily.
   b. Posterolateral dislocations occasionally cannot be reduced via closed methods and require open reduction.
3. The reduction maneuver is essentially longitudinal traction along with a reversing of the direction of the dislocation.

Indications for Use

Knee dislocation (Figure 11-13)

Precautions

1. A thorough clinical examination must be undertaken before reduction and immediately thereafter.
2. Examine the limb for motor strength, sensation, pulses, and capillary refill.
3. Altered sensation that occurs only over the dorsum of the foot suggests a neurologic injury.
4. Altered sensation in the calf and entire foot (a "stocking type" distribution) suggests a vascular injury.
5. Some surgeons recommend arterial-brachial index (ABI) measurements.
6. If the ABI is less than 0.9, then arteriography is recommended.
7. Other surgeons suggest that if a knee requires reduction, an arteriogram should be performed without regard to ABI measurement.
8. During the reduction, do not place pressure over the popliteal fossa.
9. Postreduction radiographs must be obtained.

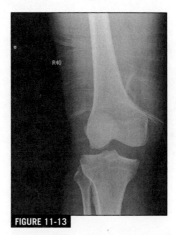

FIGURE 11-13

Pearls

A dislocated knee is a true orthopedic emergency.

Equipment

Knee immobilizer

Basic Technique

1. Patient positioning:
   a. Supine on stretcher
2. Landmarks:
   a. Patella
   b. Tibial tuberosity
   c. Femoral condyles
3. Steps:
   a. Position the patient.
   b. Obtain a physical examination.
   c. Perform a reduction.
   d. Perform a postreduction physical examination.
   e. Proceed with neurovascular management.

Detailed Technique

1. Position the patient supine on a stretcher.
2. Perform a physical examination:
   a. Check motor strength, sensation, pulses, and capillary refill.
   b. Examine the popliteal fossa for an expanding hematoma.
   c. Determine what direction the dislocation is in.
3. Perform a reduction:
   a. Stabilize the femur.
   b. Apply longitudinal traction via the tibia (Figure 11-14).

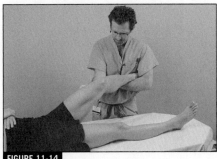

FIGURE 11-14

    c. Apply a reversing force to the direction of dislocation also via the tibia (Figure 11-15).

    d. Typically the knee will reduce.

4. Perform a postreduction physical examination.
5. Place a knee immobilizer at 15 degrees of knee flexion (Figure 11-16).
6. Proceed with neurovascular management.

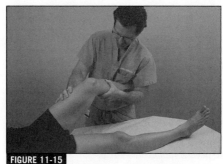

FIGURE 11-15

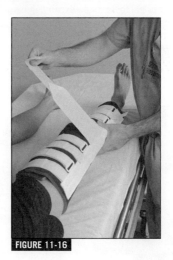

FIGURE 11-16

ANKLE FRACTURE REDUCTION

Overview

1. The majority of ankle fractures are fractures of the supination, external-rotation type.
2. The traction reduction method is based on a modification of the reduction maneuver described by Quigley.
3. The principle is to elevate the limb in such a way that the ankle falls into a pronation, internal rotation position.
4. A manual reduction technique can be performed if traction is unavailable or not desired.

Indications for Use

Supination external rotation ankle fractures (Figure 11-17) or fracture dislocations

Precautions

1. Do not use an intravenous (IV) stand attached to the ceiling unless it is specifically designed to handle large weights.
2. Ensure that the IV pole is safely secured to the bed.
3. In some cases, the IV pole can be wedged in behind the wheels of the bed.
4. In other cases, heavy tape must be used to secure the IV pole to the bed.
5. Heavy weights should be placed on the IV pole stand.

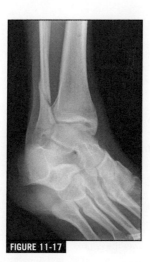

FIGURE 11-17

Pearls

1. Perform an intra-articular ankle block prior to performing this maneuver (see Chapter 7).
2. Many patients will require conscious sedation.
3. Be patient! This maneuver may require several minutes to become effective. The patient will naturally attempt to counter the forces and only time will result in muscle fatigue, causing relaxation and allowing reduction.
4. Forewarn patients that their toes may hurt more than their ankles by virtue of the toe traps. Also inform them that the toes will likely turn blue but that this symptom is normal, expected, and will resolve shortly after the toe traps are removed.

Equipment

1. If using traction:
   a. 2-inch rolled gauze
   b. IV pole
   c. Weights
2. Supplies for an AO splint (see Chapter 14)

Basic Technique: Traction

1. Patient positioning:
   a. Supine on stretcher
   b. IV pole secured at head of bed on contralateral side
2. Landmarks:
   a. Malleoli
   b. Calcaneus
3. Steps:
   a. Set up the equipment.
   b. Position the patient.
   c. Perform an intra-articular ankle block.
   d. Attach toe traps.
   e. Elevate the limb.
   f. Await reduction.
   g. Apply a splint.

Detailed Technique: Traction

1. Set up the equipment:
   a. Place an IV pole at the head of the patient's bed.
   b. The IV pole should be toward the opposite side of the injury.
   c. Securely fasten the pole to the bed either by wedging it in between the wheels and the handles or by using heavy tape.
   d. Ensure that the IV pole has the ability to be raised and lowered.
      (1) Completely lower the IV pole.
      (2) If the IV pole cannot be raised and lowered, ensure it is at a height that will allow elevation of the limb.
2. Position the patient.
3. Perform an intra-articular ankle block. Inject the ankle with lidocaine and ropivacaine (see Chapter 7).
4. Attach toe traps.

5. Attach the stockinette to your finger using a dual-ring construct:
   a. Make a loop of stockinette (Figure 11-18).
   b. Place the loop between the web space of the hallux and second toe.
   c. While holding one side of the stockinette taut, place your other hand into the loop.
   d. Spread your fingers and pull upward.
   e. Hook each side around the hallux and second toe (Figure 11-19).
   f. Pull the free end so it is taut.
6. Elevate the limb:
   a. Take the free end of the stockinette and pull it so it is taut.
   b. Secure the stockinette to the top of the IV pole.
   c. Raise the IV pole to elevate the limb (Figure 11-20).
7. Await reduction. Wait 2 to 5 minutes.
8. Apply a splint.

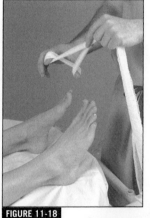

FIGURE 11-18

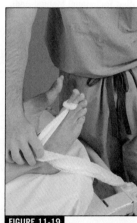

FIGURE 11-19

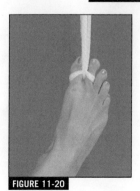

FIGURE 11-20

Basic Technique: Manual Reduction

1. Patient positioning:
   a. Supine or sitting on stretcher with the knee and lower leg off the table
2. Landmarks:
   a. Malleoli
   b. Calcaneus
3. Steps:
   a. Set up equipment.
   b. Position the patient.
   c. Perform an intra-articular ankle block.
   d. Perform a reduction maneuver if necessary.
   e. Apply a splint while an assistant holds the reduction.
   f. Apply a mold.

Detailed Technique: Manual Reduction

1. Position the patient.
2. Perform an intra-articular ankle block. Inject the ankle with lidocaine and ropivacaine (see Chapter 7).
3. Cup the heel with your hand and place your other hand on the subcutaneous portion of the mid tibia while resting the ball of the foot on your thigh (Figure 11-21); alternatively, use your forearm to maintain a plantigrade foot position (Figure 11-22).
4. Have an assistant hold the reduction by pulling up on the great toe and maintaining traction (if an assistant is not available, perform the reduction maneuver after the splint is applied but before it is set).
5. Apply an AO splint (see Chapter 14).
6. Perform a reduction maneuver as previously described to apply a mold.

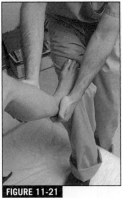

FIGURE 11-21

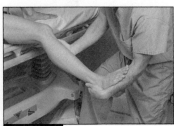
FIGURE 11-22

SUBTALAR DISLOCATION

Overview

1. Subtalar dislocations are rare and typically cause marked deformity of the foot.
2. The majority of dislocations are medial and are caused by forceful inversion of the plantarflexed foot.
3. The reduction maneuver is longitudinal traction, exaggeration of the deformity, and subsequent reversing of the direction of dislocation.

Indications for Use

Subtalar dislocation (Figures 11-23 and 11-24)

Precautions

1. Because subtalar dislocations have a high rate of associated injuries, a computed tomography scan should be obtained after the reduction.
2. Approximately one third of medial dislocations and half of lateral dislocations cannot be closed in a reduced manner. Excessive attempts at reduction should be avoided.

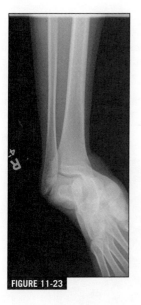

FIGURE 11-23

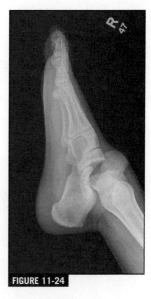

FIGURE 11-24

Pearls

1. An assistant should be used to keep the hip and knee flexed so as to relax the pull of the gastrocnemius.
2. Conscious sedation is virtually mandatory in most patients.
3. Typically, a pop or clunk signifies successful reduction.

Equipment

None

Basic Technique

1. Patient positioning:
   a. Supine on stretcher
2. Landmarks:
   a. Medial and lateral malleoli
   b. Calcaneus
3. Steps:
   a. Obtain conscious sedation.
   b. Position the patient.
   c. Perform a reduction maneuver.

Detailed Technique

1. Obtain conscious sedation.
2. Position the patient. The patient should be completely supine.
3. Perform a reduction maneuver:
   a. The patient's knee is flexed to 90 degrees and the hip is also flexed to 90 degrees by an assistant. Countertraction should be held above the ankle.
   b. Medial dislocation:
      (1) The surgeon should grasp the calcaneus with his or her dominant hand and place the opposite hand over the dorsum of the forefoot (Figure 11-25).

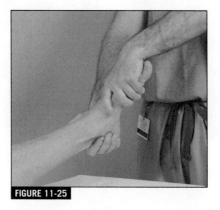

FIGURE 11-25

(2) The surgeon pulls longitudinal traction with the assistant holding countertraction.
(3) The position of the foot should be exaggerated by hyperinverting and plantarflexing the foot while maintaining longitudinal traction (Figure 11-26).
(4) The foot can then be everted and dorsiflexed to achieve reduction (Figure 11-27).

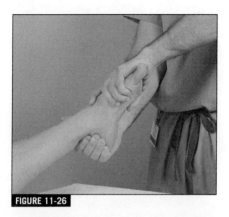

FIGURE 11-26

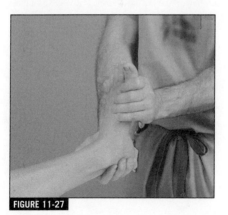

FIGURE 11-27

c. Lateral dislocation:
    (1) The surgeon should grasp the calcaneus with his or her dominant hand and place the opposite hand over the dorsum of the forefoot with a thumb over the navicular.

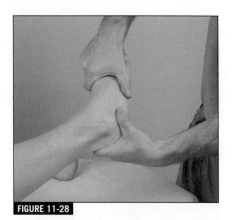

FIGURE 11-28

(2) The surgeon pulls, providing longitudinal traction, while an assistant provides countertraction.
(3) The position of the foot should be exaggerated by hypereverting and abducting the foot while maintaining longitudinal traction.
(4) The foot is inverted with plantarward and medialward pressure applied by the thumb to achieve reduction (Figure 11-28).
4. Splint the extremity with a posterior splint or an AO splint (see Chapter 14).

PART 3

SPLINTS AND CASTS

Chapter 12

Basics of Splinting and Casting

BASIC PRINCIPLES

First, Do No Harm

1. Make sure that the potential complications of applying and maintaining a cast or splint are less severe and less likely than the complications of an untreated injury.
2. A poorly made splint/cast can result in pressure sores, compression neuropathies, joint stiffness, and complex regional pain syndrome.
3. Never place a circumferential rigid dressing (cast) over an increasingly edematous limb because compartment syndrome can result.
4. Elastic bandages such as an all cotton elastic (ACE) bandage should be applied loosely so that the elasticity can accommodate any future swelling.
5. Elbows, forearms, and the lower leg and foot have the highest risk of compartment syndrome after cast application. Use caution when applying a cast in the acute setting.
6. Because plaster can expand, it is better to use plaster rather than the more rigid fiberglass cast in the acute setting.
7. Plaster and fiberglass cure with an exothermic reaction; thus inadequate padding, lack of exposure to ambient air (under a blanket), or use of water that is above room temperature can result in thermal injuries, including second-degree burns.

What to Immobilize

1. For intraarticular or periarticular fractures, the bone proximal and distal to the joint involved should be included (one above and one below).
2. For extra-articular fractures, immobilize one joint above and one joint below.
3. Immobilizing more joints than is necessary can result in permanent iatrogenic loss of joint motion.
4. Immobilization of fewer joints than is necessary can result in fracture displacement, neurovascular injury, and unnecessary pain and suffering.
5. Examples of correct immobilization:
   a. Wrist fracture (distal radius):
      (1) Bone above = the radius; begin the cast/splint above the elbow to prevent forearm (radial) rotation at the wrist.

      (2) Bone below = the carpals; end the cast/splint just proximal to the metacarpophalangeal joints (Figures 12-1 and 12-2).

  b. Tibial shaft fracture:

      (1) Joint above = the knee; begin the cast/splint as high up the leg as possible to limit knee motion.

      (2) Joint below = the ankle; end the cast/splint just proximal to the toes to limit ankle motion.

  c. Ankle fracture (distal fibula/tibia):

      (1) Bone above = the fibula + tibia; begin the cast/splint just distal to the knee joint.

      (2) Bone below = the talus; end the cast/splint just proximal to the toes.

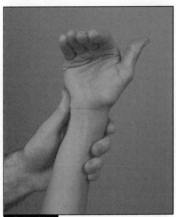

FIGURE 12-1

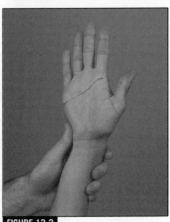

FIGURE 12-2

What Position to Immobilize

1. Unless a pressing reason exists to do otherwise, each joint should be immobilized in the optimal position to retain joint mobility after the cast/splint is removed.
2. Specific positions:
   a. Shoulder: adduction and internal rotation (Figure 12-3)
   b. Elbow: 90 degrees of flexion (see Figure 12-3)
   c. Wrist: 30 degrees of extension (Figure 12-4)
   d. Thumb: midway between maximal radial and palmar abduction (Figure 12-5)
   e. Hand: intrinsic plus (metaphalangeal joints in at least 70 degrees of flexion and interphalangeal joints in extension) (Figure 12-6)

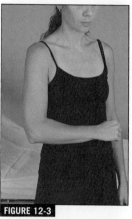

FIGURE 12-3

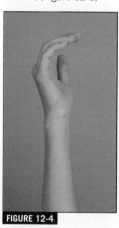

FIGURE 12-4

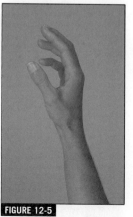

FIGURE 12-5

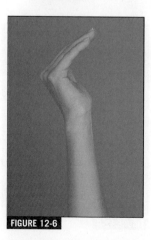

FIGURE 12-6

12

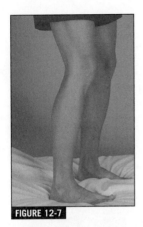

FIGURE 12-7

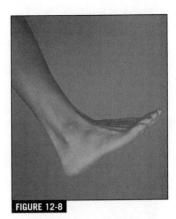

FIGURE 12-8

  f. Hip: 10 to 30 degrees of abduction, 20 to 45 degrees of flexion, 15
     degrees of external rotation
  g. Knee: 15 to 30 degrees of flexion (Figure 12-7)
  h. Ankle: neutral dorsiflexion (Figure 12-8)

Bivalving

1. If a cast is placed in the acute setting and edema is a concern, the cast
   can be split longitudinally along two sides (bivalving).
2. Splitting the cast material and the cast padding provides the most
   decompression.
3. Split the cast in a way such that divergence of the two cast "halves"
   does not compromise fracture reduction. For example, for distal radius
   fractures, split the cast directly dorsally and volarly (Figures 12-9 and
   12-10).

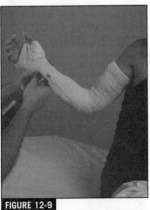

FIGURE 12-9

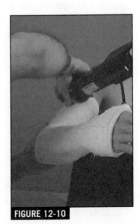

FIGURE 12-10

4. For minimal edema, a single split can be performed (monovalving).
5. After the cast is split, overwrap it with either self-adhesive or elastic bandages.

Wedging

1. If the fracture reduction is acceptable in translation but not in angulation, the cast can be cut transversely on the acute angle of the malreduction and a wedge inserted to change the angle of the cast (Figure 12-11).
2. Because it is difficult to calculate the size of the wedge, it is best to apply a temporary wedge while radiographs are taken, followed by definitive wedge placement. Tongue depressors can be used as temporary wedges (Figure 12-12).
3. Wedges should be made out of plaster even if the cast is fiberglass (Figures 12-13 and 12-14).
4. Overwrap with the same material as the remainder of the cast (Figure 12-15).

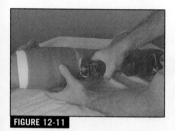

FIGURE 12-11

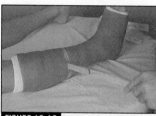

FIGURE 12-12

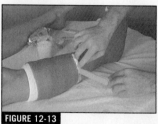

FIGURE 12-13

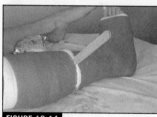

FIGURE 12-14

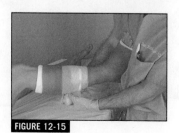

FIGURE 12-15

Cast Removal

1. Overview
   a. A cast saw is an oscillating saw designed to cut hard cast material while minimizing trauma to soft material, such as cotton padding and skin.
      (1) The oscillations generate significant heat and can easily burn a patient.
      (2) Approximately 1% of cast removals are associated with a cast saw burn (Figure 12-16).
   b. A cast saw is necessary for removal of fiberglass casts (Figure 12-17).
   c. Plaster casts can be unraveled after they are soaked in water for several minutes; however, finding the leading end of the plaster strip can be difficult.
   d. Do not attempt to place any cast if a cast saw is not available, because emergent removal or trimming of the cast may be necessary.
   e. A cast spreader can be very helpful in separating the two halves of a cast after they have been split (Figure 12-18).

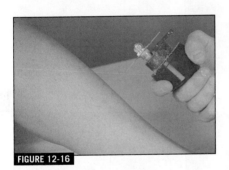
FIGURE 12-16

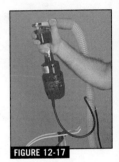
FIGURE 12-17

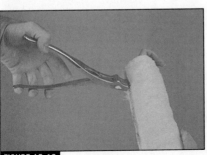
FIGURE 12-18

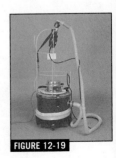
FIGURE 12-19

f. We recommend that a cast saw be attached to suction to limit the volume of aerosolized particulate debris on clothes and in your lungs (Figure 12-19).

g. Removal of waterproof casts is associated with a higher risk of cast saw burns because the padding is less heat resistant and thinner than is conventional cast padding.

2. Technique

   a. It is important to use an "up, over, down" technique when cutting a cast.

   b. The cast saw should be pushed directly down into the cast (Figure 12-20). Your index finger should rest on the cast to limit the excursion of the cast saw.

   c. The saw should then be removed by coming straight back up.

   d. The saw should then be moved longitudinally to the next point on the cast.

   e. The saw is then reinserted using the same technique.

   f. Intermittently check the temperature of the blade. The blade can be cooled with an alcohol wipe.

   g. *Never drag the cast saw along the cast.* This technique significantly increases the risk of a cut or a burn.

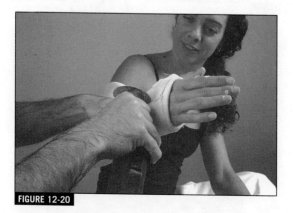

FIGURE 12-20

MATERIALS

Stockinette

1. Stockinettes are available in 1- to 6-inch widths and in rolls of several yards in length.
2. Stockinettes may be used as a border to provide a more finished appearance to casts (Figure 12-21).
3. Stockinettes may be used for traction set-up (Figure 12-22).

Cast Padding

1. Cast padding is available in cotton, synthetic, and waterproof varieties and in sizes ranging from 1 to 6 inches (Figure 12-23).

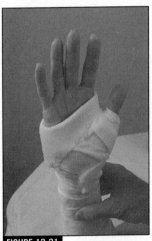

FIGURE 12-21

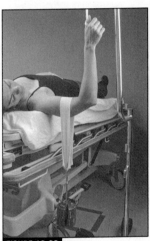

FIGURE 12-22

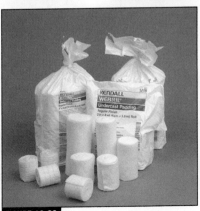

FIGURE 12-23

2. We prefer the cotton variety of cast padding because it expands more evenly, is more comfortable, and is easier to work with compared with other varieties.
3. Use cast padding to provide a cuff between the casting material and the skin.
4. Avoid placing a seam of cast padding or too much padding material on the flexion side of a joint, because pressure ulcers can result (Figure 12-24).
5. Avoid wrinkles and creases in the cast padding, which can result in pressure ulcers (Figure 12-25).

Plaster

1. Plaster is available in sizes ranging from 1- to 6-inch-wide rolls and strips (Figure 12-26).
2. The plaster content and quality of the rolls and strips varies by manufacturer.

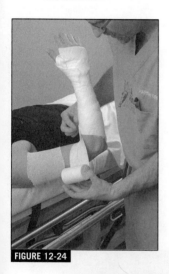

FIGURE 12-24

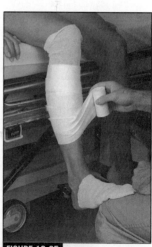

FIGURE 12-25

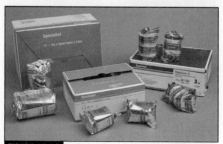

FIGURE 12-26

3. We prefer Gypsona because it has a high plaster content, makes a nice, smooth finish on the outside, and feels silky to apply.
4. Plaster can be used for any splint or cast.
5. Plaster holds a mold better than fiberglass does and is the material of choice when a reduction is required.
6. Plaster expands more than fiberglass and is better suited to the acute setting.
7. Unlike fiberglass, plaster loses all structural integrity in water and must be kept dry.
8. A plaster splint/cast will take 24 hours to fully cure.
9. Avoid air pockets or bubbles in the plaster, which form a stress riser inside the cast and lead to structural failure.
10. Avoid direct contact between the skin and plaster, which can result in abrasions and lacerations.

Fiberglass

1. Fiberglass is available in a variety of sizes and colors ranging from 1 to 6 inches and from hot pink to army green (Figure 12-27).
2. Fiberglass takes just a few minutes to reach near full structural integrity and is more resistant to deformation than is plaster. Because of these qualities, molding with fiberglass is much more difficult than molding with plaster.
3. Water does not compromise a fiberglass cast, and waterproof cast padding can be used if a patient intends to go in the water or if it is suspected he or she will do so.
4. Fiberglass can be used to hold a nondisplaced fracture in position.
5. Use cut-to-length fiberglass splints with caution:
   a. Pad the edges (which can be as sharp as cut glass).
   b. Use the correct width.
   c. Place the padded side toward the skin.
6. Be sure to wring out any excess moisture from the fiberglass after activating it in water to prevent maceration of the cast padding.
7. Do not use a fiberglass cast in the acute setting unless the patient will be under close observation in the hospital, and never use it in the acute setting on an obtunded patient.

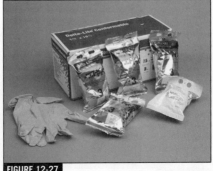

FIGURE 12-27

8. Avoid direct contact between the skin and fiberglass, which can result in abrasions and lacerations.
9. Fiberglass that is colored can leave a stain on clothes or skin.

Elastic Cast Material

1. Elastic cast material is available in sizes ranging from 1 to 3 inches.
2. We use 3M Soft cast (Figure 12-28).
3. Elastic cast material can be used for young children who do not require rigid immobilization and are unlikely to tolerate cast removal with a saw.
4. Avoid using elastic cast material if a reduction was attempted.
5. Avoid direct contact between the skin and elastic cast material, which can result in abrasions and lacerations.

Elastic Bandage

1. Elastic bandages are available in a variety of sizes and colors ranging from 2 to 6 inches and from hot pink to army green (Figure 12-29).

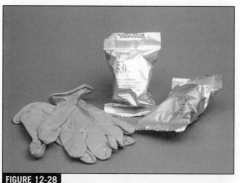

FIGURE 12-28

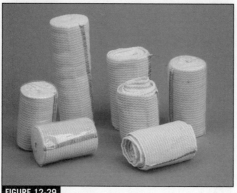

FIGURE 12-29

2. The first elastic bandage was developed in 1914 and was termed an ACE (all cotton elastic) bandage.
3. Use elastic bandages to overwrap splints or bivalved casts.
4. Use larger sizes for a swath.
5. Use elastic bandages for bulky Jones dressings.
6. Avoid applying the bandage under tension; the elasticity is intended to accommodate swelling.
7. Avoid applying more than two layers of elastic bandage (50% overlap) to allow swelling.

Self-Adherent Bandage

1. Self-adherent bandages are available in a variety of sizes and colors ranging from 1 to 6 inches and from hot pink to army green (Figure 12-30).
2. Self-adherent bandages are available as Coban and Co-Flex.
3. Use self-adherent bandages to overwrap splints or bivalved casts.
4. Use larger sizes for a swath.
5. We prefer to use self-adherent bandages rather than elastic-type bandages for the following reasons:
   a. They have a better cosmetic appearance.
   b. They are less likely to overtighten.
   c. They are harder for patient to remove.
   d. They wear better over time.
6. Avoid applying the bandage under tension; the elasticity is intended to accommodate swelling.
7. Avoid applying more than two layers of self-adherent bandages (50% overlap) to allow swelling.

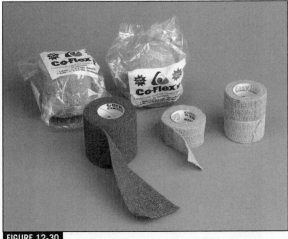

FIGURE 12-30

SPLINT PRODUCTION BASICS

Padding

1. Application of cast padding:
   a. Begin with a circumferential wrap at one end (Figure 12-31).
   b. Progress to the other end while overlapping each layer by 50% (Figure 12-32).
   c. Return to the starting point while overlapping each layer by 50%.
   d. Avoid seams on the concave side of a joint: "span the fossa" (Figure 12-33).
2. Avoid wrinkles (see Figure 12-25).
3. Application of cast padding cuffs (Figure 12-34):

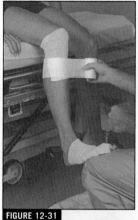

FIGURE 12-31

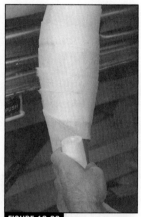

FIGURE 12-32

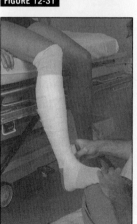

FIGURE 12-33

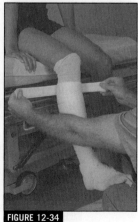

FIGURE 12-34

a. A two-ply cuff of cast padding is applied at the terminal portions of a cast.
b. Typically, a piece of cast padding is folded onto itself (Figure 12-35):
   (1) This technique creates a loose end and a folded end, with a small tear starting at the loose end to get around corners if necessary (Figure 12-36).
   (2) The folded end is always positioned toward the outside of the cast (Figure 12-37).

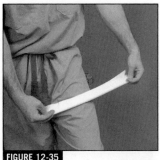

FIGURE 12-35

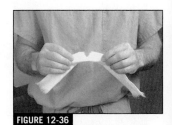

FIGURE 12-36

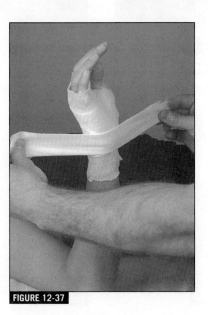

FIGURE 12-37

Types of Splints

1. Plaster onlay splint (Figure 12-38):
   a. The cast padding is applied to the limb, then the slab of plaster is laid onto the cast padding.
   b. Cast padding is then rolled over the plaster.
   c. This technique produces the best conforming and most versatile splint.
2. Plaster prepadded splint (Figure 12-39):
   a. Instead of placing cast padding directly on the limb, a splint can be prepadded and applied as a unit.
   b. A plaster prepadded splint is best for coaptation splints.
   c. Commercial prepadded plaster splint material is available.
   d. Prepadded plaster splint material can be placed inside a stockinette for additional versatility.
3. Fiberglass prepadded splint:
   a. A fiberglass prepadded splint is a strip of fiberglass inside cast padding material that can be cut to any desired length.
   b. Commercially made fiberglass prepadded splints are available in a variety of widths from 3 to 6 inches. *We do not recommend use of this type of product.*

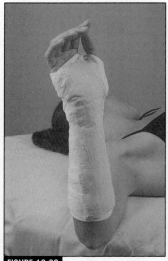

FIGURE 12-38

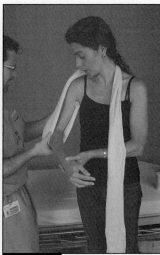

FIGURE 12-39

Plaster Onlay Splint

1. Place two layers of cast padding to allow a 1- to 2-cm cuff of padding proximal and distal to the plaster (Figure 12-40).
2. Measure out the correct length of splinting material (Figure 12-41). Keep in mind that plaster will shrink in water by approximately 5%.
3. Prepare 10 to 12 layers of splinting material of the measured length and adequate width (Figure 12-42).
4. Activate the plaster by placing it in tepid water.
5. Allow the plaster to soak until it is softened (Figure 12-43).

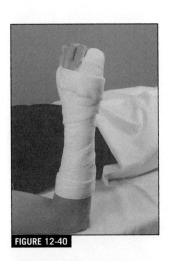
FIGURE 12-40

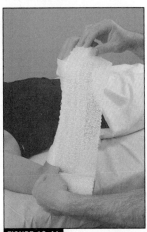
FIGURE 12-41

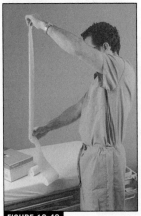
FIGURE 12-42

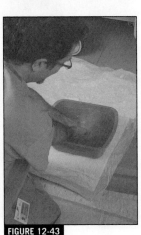
FIGURE 12-43

6. Remove any excess moisture from the plaster (Figure 12-44).
7. Wring any air pockets or bubbles out of the plaster by running the strip between two fingers (Figures 12-45 and 12-46).
8. Apply the plaster slab to the limb.
9. If the slab is too long, either fold it back (Figure 12-47) or cut it to size (Figure 12-48).

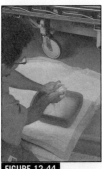
FIGURE 12-44

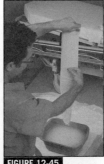
FIGURE 12-45

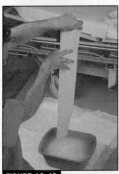
FIGURE 12-46

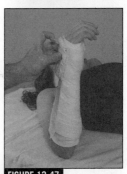
FIGURE 12-47

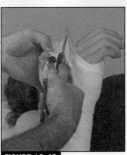
FIGURE 12-48

12

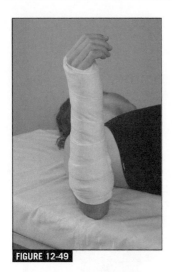

FIGURE 12-49

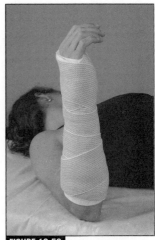

FIGURE 12-50

10. Overwrap with cast padding (Figure 12-49).
11. Overwrap with an elastic or self-adherent bandage (Figure 12-50).

Plaster Prepadded Splint

1. Measure out the correct length of splinting material (Figure 12-51). Keep in mind that plaster will shrink in water by approximately 5%.
2. Prepare 10 to 12 layers of splinting material of the measured length and adequate width (Figure 12-52).

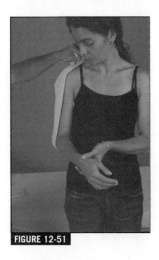

FIGURE 12-51

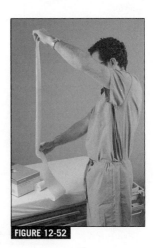

FIGURE 12-52

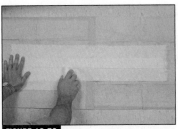
FIGURE 12-53

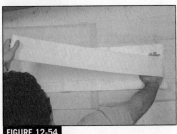
FIGURE 12-54

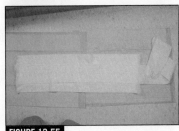
FIGURE 12-55

3. Roll out four layers of cast padding on a flat surface a few centimeters longer than and twice as wide as the slab of plaster (Figure 12-53).
4. Place a strip of cast padding twice the length of the plaster slab in the center of the cast padding (12-54 and 12-55).
5. Activate the plaster by placing it in tepid water.
6. Allow the plaster to soak until it is softened (see Figure 12-43).
7. Remove any excess moisture from the plaster (see Figure 12-44).
8. Wring any air pockets or bubbles out of the plaster by running the strip between two fingers (see Figures 12-45 and 12-46).
9. Place the plaster slab in the center of the padding material (Figure 12-56).

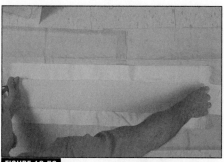

FIGURE 12-56

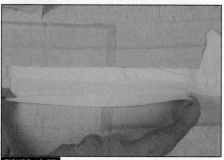

FIGURE 12-57

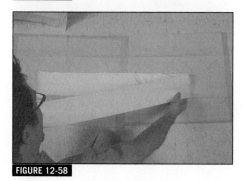

FIGURE 12-58

10. Fold over the cast padding to cover the edges of the plaster slab (Figure 12-57).
11. Fold a double-length strip of padding to cover any exposed plaster (Figure 12-58).
12. Place the splint into a stockinette for extra padding if desired (Figure 12-59).

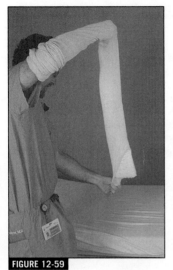

FIGURE 12-59

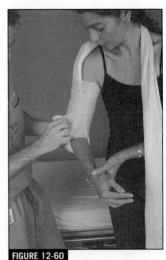

FIGURE 12-60

13. Apply the prepadded splint to the limb (see Figure 12-39).
14. If the splint material is too long, either fold it back or cut it to size.
15. Overwrap the splint with an elastic or self-adherent bandage
    (Figure 12-60).

Fiberglass Prepadded Splint

1. Place two layers of cast padding to allow a 1- to 2-cm cuff of padding
   proximal and distal to the plaster.
2. Measure out the correct length of splinting material.
3. Cut the splint to size.
4. Ensure that no fiberglass is exposed at the cut ends.
5. Activate the fiberglass by placing it in tepid water.
6. Remove any excess moisture from the fiberglass.
7. Apply the prepadded splint to the limb.
8. If the splint material is too long, either fold it back or cut it to size.
9. Overwrap the splint with an elastic or self-adherent bandage.

12

CAST PRODUCTION BASICS

Types of Casts

1. Plaster cast:
   a. The strength of the cast depends on the removal of any air pockets from between each sheet of plaster.
      (1) Use very wet plaster.
      (2) Always roll the plaster on the cast. Do not lift the roll of plaster away from the cast (Figure 12-61); a "wall" of liquid plaster will form between the roll and the cast and help fill in air spaces.
      (3) Be sure to laminate (i.e., smooth plaster into any remaining air pockets) as you roll each layer of the cast (Figures 12-62, 12-63, and 12-64).

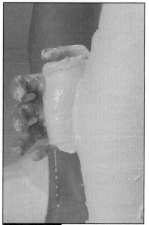

FIGURE 12-61

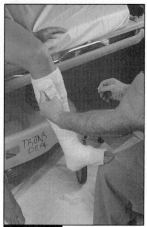

FIGURE 12-62

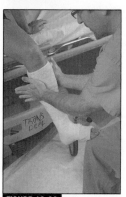

FIGURE 12-63

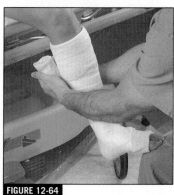

FIGURE 12-64

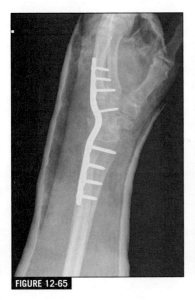

FIGURE 12-65

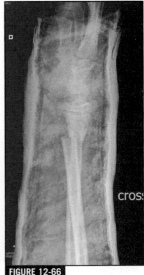

cros

FIGURE 12-66

    (4) A well-made cast needs to be only four to six layers thick.

    (5) Look at your plaster on postreduction radiographs: the plaster should be one solid line with no onion-skinning appearance (Figure 12-65).

    (6) A badly made cast will have uneven plaster thickness, show "onion skinning," and appear fuzzy (Figure 12-66).

  b. Advantages of a plaster cast:

    (1) A plaster cast will accommodate a small amount of edema.

    (2) A plaster cast is the best mode of immobilization to hold a fracture reduction.

  c. Disadvantages of a plaster cast:

    (1) Even a well-made plaster cast will begin to crumble after 6 weeks and may need to be reinforced with a fiberglass outer shell.

    (2) Creating a plaster cast is technically more demanding.

    (3) Creating a plaster cast is messy.

2. Fiberglass cast:
   a. Fiberglass should be rolled away from the skin (Figure 12-67).
      (1) Avoid placing too much tension on the fiberglass.
      (2) Be careful with any exposed edges on skin.
   b. Advantages of a fiberglass cast:
      (1) A fiberglass cast will retain its structural integrity in water.
      (2) A fiberglass cast comes in colors.
      (3) A fiberglass cast is lightweight yet strong.
      (4) A fiberglass cast is easier to apply than a plaster cast.
   c. Disadvantages of a fiberglass cast:
      (1) A fiberglass cast will not hold a fracture reduction.
      (2) A fiberglass cast will not expand to accommodate any swelling.
3. Elastic cast:
   a. Elastic casting material should be rolled away from the skin.
      (1) Avoid placing too much tension on the elastic material.
      (2) Be careful with any exposed edges on skin.
   b. Advantages of elastic casting material:
      (1) Elastic casting material will retain its structural integrity in water.
      (2) Elastic casting material is lightweight.
      (3) Elastic casting material allows some motion.
      (4) Elastic casting material is easier to apply than a plaster cast.
   c. Disadvantages of elastic casting material:
      (1) Elastic casting material will not hold a fracture reduction.
      (2) Elastic casting material will not expand to accommodate any swelling.
      (3) Elastic casting material allows some motion.

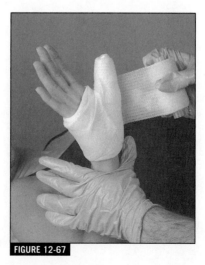

FIGURE 12-67

Plaster Cast

1. Cut two pieces of stockinette, one for the proximal end and one for the distal end.
2. Place the stockinette onto the limb (Figure 12-68).
3. Place two layers of cast padding to allow a 1- to 2-cm cuff of padding proximal and distal to the plaster (Figure 12-69).
4. Fold back the stockinette to create a neat edge (Figure 12-70).

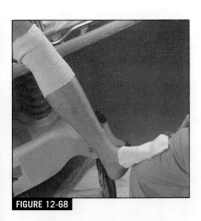

FIGURE 12-68

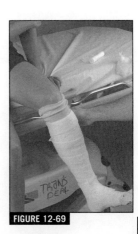

FIGURE 12-69

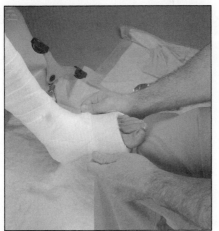

FIGURE 12-70

5. Activate the plaster by placing it in tepid water.
6. Allow the plaster to soak until it is softened (Figure 12-71).
7. Do not wring out the plaster: keep it sloppy wet (Figure 12-72).
8. Apply the plaster to the limb.
   a. Begin with a circumferential wrap at one end.
   b. Progress to the other end while overlapping each layer by 50%.
   c. Return to the starting point while overlapping each layer by 50%.
   d. Avoid seams on the concave side of a joint: "span the fossa" (Figure 12-73).
9. If the plaster encroaches on the cuff of the cast padding or is in contact with the skin, wait until it has cured (5 to 10 minutes) and then trim it with a cast saw.

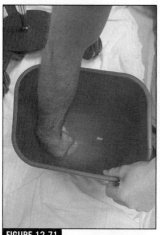

FIGURE 12-71

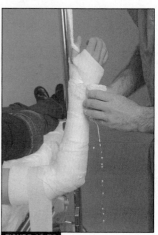

FIGURE 12-72

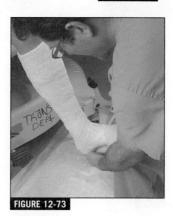

FIGURE 12-73

10. Tips and tricks:
    a. Around elbows, knees, and ankles, apply a four-layer plaster slab to the convex side of the joint to minimize bulk on the concave side.
    b. Roll four times around either end of the cast to ensure that both ends are rigid.
    c. To laminate the cast as you go, smooth out the plaster with the hand not holding the plaster roll.
        (1) While pulling the roll of plaster toward you with your right hand, the left hand should mirror that motion while pressing the heel of your hand against the cast (see Figure 12-63).
        (2) While pushing the roll of plaster away from you with your left hand, the right hand should mirror that motion while pressing the heel of your hand against the cast (Figure 12-74).
    d. To get around the thumb-index web space, either twist the roll 360 degrees or pinch the sheet of plaster (Figures 12-75 and 12-76).

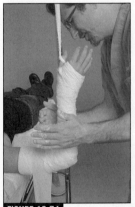

FIGURE 12-74

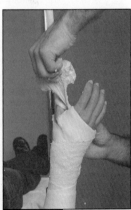

FIGURE 12-75

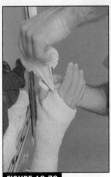

FIGURE 12-76

e. To make a turn:
   (1) Lift the plaster away from the limb.
   (2) Pinch one end of the strip (Figure 12-77).
   (3) Angle the plaster and begin the roll (Figure 12-78).
   (4) Smooth out (laminate) the dog ear (Figures 12-79 and 12-80).
f. When the roll of plaster begins to unravel, it is called a "banana."

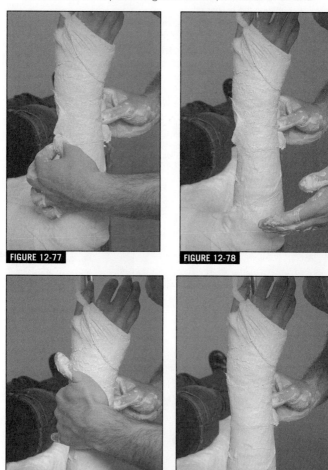

FIGURE 12-77

FIGURE 12-78

FIGURE 12-79

FIGURE 12-80

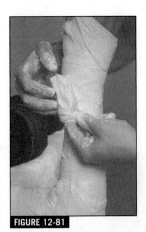

FIGURE 12-81

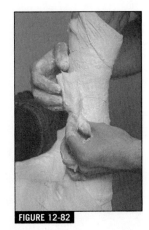

FIGURE 12-82

(1) If a banana occurs, push the plaster back in and pinch the end closed (Figures 12-81 and 12-82).
(2) If a banana cannot be fixed, cut off the roll and begin a new roll.

Fiberglass/Elastic Cast

1. Cut two pieces of stockinette, one for the proximal end and one for the distal end.
2. Place the stockinette onto the arm.
3. Place two layers of cast padding to allow a 1- to 2-cm cuff of padding proximal and distal to the cast material.
4. Fold back the stockinette to create a neat edge.
5. Activate the cast material by placing it in tepid water.
6. Remove any excess moisture from the casting material (Figure 12-83).

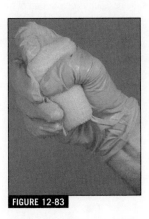

FIGURE 12-83

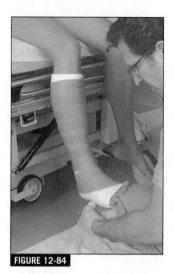

FIGURE 12-84

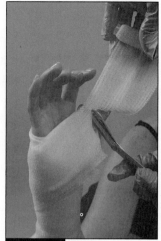

FIGURE 12-85

7. Apply the casting material to the limb.
   a. Begin with a circumferential wrap at one end.
   b. Progress to the other end while overlapping each layer by 50%.
   c. Return to the starting point while overlapping each layer by 50%.
   d. Avoid seams on the concave side of a joint: "span the fossa" (Figure 12-84).
   e. The casting material can be cut with trauma shears to facilitate turns and passage through web spaces (Figure 12-85).
8. If the casting material encroaches on the cuff of the cast padding or is in contact with the skin, wait until it has cured (5 to 10 minutes) and then trim it with a cast saw.

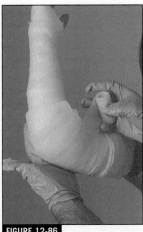

FIGURE 12-86

9. Tips and tricks:
   a. Around elbows, knees, and ankles, shuffle the casting material back and forth over the convex side of the joint to minimize bulk on the concave side (Figure 12-86).
   b. Roll four times around either end of the cast to ensure that both ends are rigid.

COMMON ERRORS

1. Padding is inappropriate:
   a. Too little padding can lead to pressure necrosis and saw burns.
   b. Too much padding can result in inadequate immobilization and does not accommodate swelling.
   c. Wrinkled padding can cause pressure necrosis.
2. Activating plaster in hot water:
   a. Casting material often is activated in hot water to reduce the amount of time needed for the cast to harden.
   b. The faster casting material sets, the more heat is produced.
   c. Heat produced by fast-setting casting material places the patient at risk for thermal injury.
3. Cast material thickness too thick:
   a. The more material that is used, the larger the exothermic reaction and the greater the risk of thermal injury.

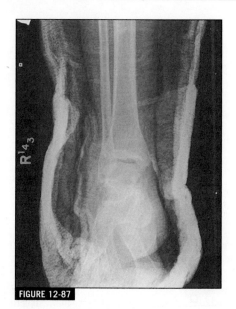

FIGURE 12-87

4. Failure to allow the splint or cast to fully harden:
   a. A busy clinician may leave a recently applied splint or cast on a pillow or on a stretcher.
   b. Static pressure from the pillow or stretcher can increase the temperature at that pressure point, leading to thermal injury.
   c. Any molding may be lost if the casting material has not hardened. This consequence most commonly occurs when applying a splint or cast around the ankle; as a result, the foot falls into equinus.
5. The cast is wrapped too tightly:
   a. COMPARTMENT SYNDROME!
6. The cast or splint is applied unevenly:
   a. The tendency exists to apply more of the splint around the apex of the injury.
   b. An unevenly applied cast or splint is most commonly detected on postapplication radiographs (Figure 12-87).

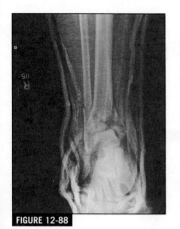

FIGURE 12-88

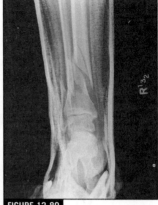

FIGURE 12-89

7. The cast or splint is not laminated:
   a. Lack of lamination results in a weak splint or cast.
   b. Lack of lamination is most commonly detected on postapplication radiographs as an onion-skinning appearance (Figure 12-88). The plaster should be one solid line (Figure 12-89).
8. The wrong joints are immobilized or the joints are immobilized in the wrong position:
   a. Immobilizing more joints than is necessary can result in permanent iatrogenic loss of joint motion.
   b. Immobilization of fewer joints than is necessary can result in fracture displacement, neurovascular injury, and unnecessary pain and suffering.
   c. Immobilization in an incorrect position can result in both fracture displacement and iatrogenic loss of joint motion.
9. The cast saw is used in an inappropriate fashion:
   a. The cast saw should never be dragged along a cast.

12

Chapter 13

Upper Extremity Splints and Casts

FIGURE-OF-8 SPLINT

Overview

1. Figure-of-8 splints are used primarily for fractures about the clavicle.
2. Figure-of-8 splints are commercially prepared devices intended to create a reduction force on the clavicle.
3. No difference in outcome is seen between a figure-of-8 splint and a sling for closed management of clavicle fractures.

Indications for Use

1. Minimally displaced clavicle shaft fractures
2. Medial physeal clavicle fractures

Precautions

1. Closed reductions cannot be maintained and should not be attempted.
2. Avoid overtightening the splint; excessive tension can result in increased pain, compression of the axillary vessels, and brachial plexus neuropathy.

Pearls

1. Reduction is not required for most clavicle fractures.
2. Clavicle fractures with more than 1.5cm of overlap result in long-term disability and should be treated with an open reduction and internal fixation.
3. Fractures that tent the skin can erode through the skin and are unlikely to heal without open reduction and internal fixation.

Equipment

Figure-of-8 splint

Basic Technique

1. Patient positioning:
   a. Standing
2. Landmarks:
   a. Clavicle
   b. Acromioclavicular joint
3. Steps:
   a. Have the patient stand.
   b. Fit the patient with a figure-of-8 splint.
   c. The figure-of-8 splint should be placed so that the center of the "8" rests on upper back.

Detailed Technique

1. Have the patient stand (Figure 13-1).
2. Apply the figure-of-8 splint so that the center of the "8" comes to rest between the shoulder blades on the upper back (Figure 13-2).
3. Adjust the figure-of-8 dressing so that it is as tight as possible while still being comfortable to wear (Figures 13-3 and 13-4).

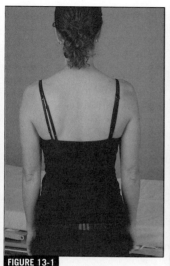

FIGURE 13-1

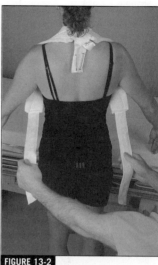

FIGURE 13-2

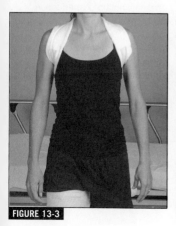

FIGURE 13-3

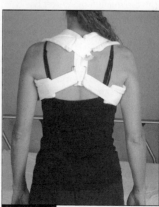

FIGURE 13-4

13

ARM SLING/ARM SLING AND SWATH

Overview

"Though simple in form and principle, this sling is rich in security, ease, and comfort."—*W.C. Wermuth, MD, 1908*

1. The arm sling is used for a variety of conditions.
2. A swath wrapped around the body is added for shoulder immobilization.

Indications for Use

1. Sling:
   a. Clavicle fractures
   b. Minimally displaced proximal humerus fractures
   c. Acromioclavicular separations
   d. Support for splints and casts of the upper extremity
2. Sling and swath: moderately displaced proximal humerus fractures where the humerus does not move as a single unit

Precautions

1. Ensure a proper fit to prevent pressure complications at the back of the neck. It is recommended that a well-padded sling be used or that the neck be padded with cast padding and/or an Army Battle Dressing (ABD) pad.
2. Elderly patients and patients with compromised skin (such as persons taking steroids on a long-term basis) should be monitored closely for skin breakdown.

Pearls

1. The adult elbow does not tolerate immobilization well. If possible given the nature of the injury, the patient should be instructed to perform daily elbow, wrist, and hand range-of-motion exercises.
2. If a reduction maneuver has been performed, obtain postreduction radiographs while the patient is wearing the sling or the sling and swath to ensure maintenance of the reduction.

Equipment

1. Arm sling or sling and swath
2. Cast padding or ABD pad
3. Talcum powder (optional)

Improvisation

An arm sling and 6-inch elastic bandage can be used if a commercial sling and swath are not available.

Basic Technique

1. Patient positioning:
   a. Standing
2. Landmarks:
   a. Clavicle
   b. Acromioclavicular joint
   c. Acromion

3. Steps:
   a. Sling:
      (1) Have the patient stand.
      (2) Fit the patient with a sling.
      (3) The sling should provide support for the weight of the arm.
   b. Sling and swath:
      (1) Have the patient stand.
      (2) Place an ABD pad with talcum powder (optional) in the axilla.
      (3) Fit the patient with a sling.
      (4) Apply the swath.

Detailed Technique

1. Sling:
   a. Have the patient stand.
   b. Pad the neck strap of the sling to prevent pressure complications at the back of the neck (Figures 13-5 and 13-6).
   c. Apply the sling and adjust the straps.
   d. Adjust the sling so it is tight enough to support the weight of the arm (Figure 13-7).

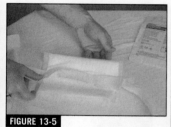

FIGURE 13-5

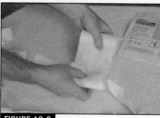

FIGURE 13-6

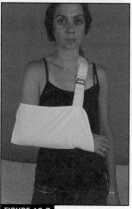

FIGURE 13-7

2. Sling and swath:
   a. Have the patient stand.
   b. Pad the neck strap of the sling to prevent pressure complications at the back of the neck.
   c. Place talcum powder on the ABD pad and fold the pad in half, with the talcum side facing out (Figure 13-8).
   d. Place the folded ABD pad in the axilla to absorb perspiration.
   e. Apply the sling and adjust the straps so it is loose while providing some support for the weight of the arm.
   f. Buckle and adjust the circumferential body strap (Figure 13-9).
   g. If using a sling only, swath the arm to the body using cast padding (Figure 13-10) followed by application of a large elastic bandage (Figure 13-11).

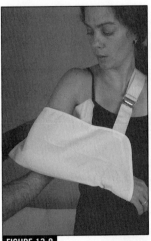

FIGURE 13-8

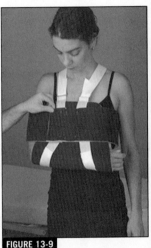

FIGURE 13-9

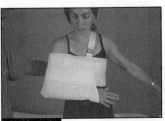

FIGURE 13-10

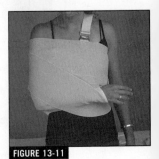

FIGURE 13-11

COAPTATION SPLINT

Overview

1. The correct application of either of the methods described below will ensure that the coaptation splint remains secure and does not fall out of place.
2. See Chapter 9 for a discussion on reduction of humeral shaft fractures.

Indications for Use

Humeral shaft fracture

Precautions

1. Do not allow one end of the coaptation splint to end at the fracture site; otherwise, the splint terminus will become a fulcrum and cause more displacement.
2. An ABD pad can be placed in the axilla after the splint is applied (see Figure 13-8).
   a. Use of an ABD pad prevents direct compression of the brachial plexus.
   b. An ABD pad absorbs moisture.
3. When using the hanging stockinette modification technique, pay close attention to which side of the splint is padded. Ensure that the well-padded side is facing toward the patient.

Pearls

1. Coaptation splints have a reputation for being made poorly and for sliding down the arm.
2. The key to applying a coaptation splint properly is to ensure that the splint always comes above the arm onto the shoulder (Figure 13-12).

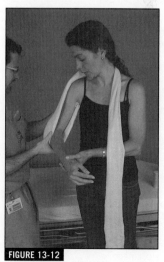

FIGURE 13-12

3. Use a technique that allows the coaptation splint to be secured around the body to prevent distal displacement. An extra-long elastic or self-adherent bandage is a useful adjunct for a coaptation splint.
4. When applying the splint, have the patient turn his or her head to the contralateral side, which prevents the neck from pushing down the splint during application.
5. We prefer using a self-adhesive bandage to overwrap the plaster because it acts predictably during application, stays in place well, and looks better than other options.

Equipment
1. Stockinette: 4 inches wide, 6 feet long
2. Cast padding: 4 inches wide
3. Plaster: 4 inches wide
4. Elastic or self-adherent bandage: 4 inches wide
5. Silk tape: 2 inches wide (optional)
6. Bucket of tepid water

Basic Technique
1. Patient positioning:
   a. If possible, have the patient stand or sit up with his or her back off the stretcher.
   b. The elbow is placed at 90 degrees.
   c. If the patient is unable to sit up, move the head of bed upright as possible.
2. Where to start:
   a. As high into the axilla as possible
   b. If the fracture is in the proximal third of the humeral diaphysis (right at the level of the axilla on the radiograph), start the splint lower.
3. Where to finish:
   a. At the base of the neck
4. Where to mold:
   a. Lateral aspect, distal to the fracture site
5. Steps:
   a. Measure the length of the splint using plaster.
   b. Roll out the cast padding.
   c. Roll out the plaster.
   d. Cut a 6-foot length of 4-inch stockinette.
   e. Position the patient.
   f. Prepare the plaster in the usual fashion.
   g. Place a splint inside a stockinette.
   h. Apply the splint.
   i. Definitively secure the splint with an elastic bandage.
   j. Complete the stockinette.

Detailed Technique

1. Measure the length of the splint.
   a. Use the contralateral side.
   b. Hold one hand in the axilla and wrap the plaster around the elbow until the base of the neck is reached.
   c. Mark the length on the plaster by making a small tear on one side.
2. Roll out the plaster (Figure 13-13).
   a. The plaster slab should be 10 to 12 sheets thick.
   b. Use the measured length.
3. Roll out the cast padding (Figure 13-14).
   a. Use the usual technique that will allow the cast padding to be folded over (see Chapter 12).
   b. Add at least 6 inches of length so the splint may be folded over.
4. Cut a 6-foot length of 4-inch stockinette.
5. Position the patient (Figure 13-15).
   a. Have the patient sit upright if possible.
   b. Place the patient's elbow at 90 degrees.
   c. Ensure that the patient's head is facing toward the contralateral side.

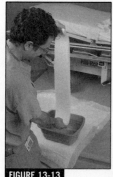

FIGURE 13-13

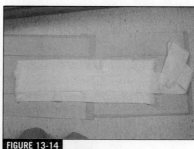

FIGURE 13-14

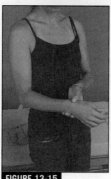

FIGURE 13-15

6. Prepare the plaster in the usual fashion (Figures 13-16 and 13-17). Use the usual technique of wetting and laminating, followed by placement in cast padding (see Chapter 12).
7. Place the splint inside a stockinette (Figure 13-18).
   a. Initially placing the entire length of the stockinette on the surgeon's forearm is helpful.
   b. Hold one end of the splint with the arm containing the stockinette.
   c. Pull the stockinette to the end of the splint.
   d. Do not forget which side of the splint is padded!
8. Apply the splint (see Figure 13-12).
   a. Start in the axilla or at an appropriate starting point given the fracture site. Provisionally secure it with cast padding at the middle arm.

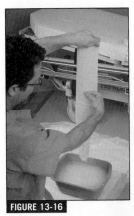

FIGURE 13-16

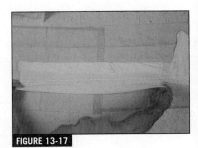

FIGURE 13-17

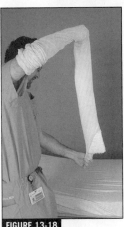

FIGURE 13-18

   b. Loop the splint around the elbow. Again, provisionally secure it with cast padding at the middle arm.

   c. Momentarily fold the remaining part of the splint down.

   d. Pass the loose end of the stockinette around the neck.

9. Definitively secure the splint with an elastic or self-adherent bandage (Figure 13-19).

   a. Wrap the elastic or self-adherent bandage around the arm and splint.

   b. Having an assistant support the arm and/or the splint can be helpful.

10. Apply the mold. Most fractures require a two-point mold, with one hand anterolateral at the fracture site and the other posteromedial at the elbow (Figure 13-20).

11. Complete the stockinette (Figures 13-21 and 13-22):

   a. Tie a slip knot in the loose end of the stockinette (an overhand knot with a draw-loop).

   b. Place the wrist of the affected side inside the slip knot to create a collar-and-cuff type construct.

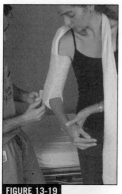
FIGURE 13-19

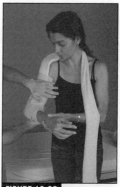
FIGURE 13-20

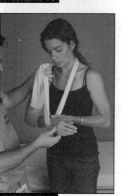
FIGURE 13-21

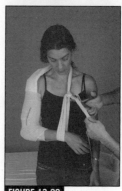
FIGURE 13-22

13

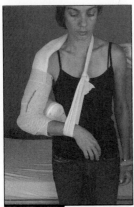

FIGURE 13-23

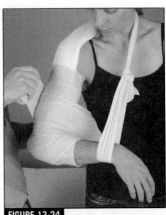

FIGURE 13-24

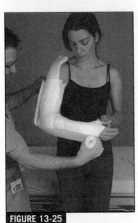

FIGURE 13-25

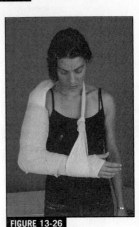

FIGURE 13-26

12. Place a cast padding wedge under the arm to counteract varus displacement of the fracture (optional) (Figures 13-23 and 13-24).
13. A posterior slab may be added to control elbow motion for more distal fractures (Figures 13-25 and 13-26).

POSTERIOR ELBOW SPLINT

Overview

1. A posterior elbow splint is inherently weak. Struts must be added to prevent elbow extension in the splint.
2. Two techniques are described for stabilization of the posterior elbow splint:
   a. External struts with tape
   b. Internal struts with plaster

Indications for Use

1. Fractures about the elbow
2. Postoperative/postinjury elbow immobilization
3. Elbow dislocations

Precautions

1. The wrist is usually immobilized to control for pronation and supination about the elbow. Elbow dislocations should be splinted in at least 90 degrees of flexion with the wrist in pronation.
2. Ensure that the splint remains proximal to the palmar flexion crease to preserve complete finger range of motion.
3. At the antecubital fossa, do not allow edges of cast padding to lay immediately within the fossa borders.
   a. Allowing edges of cast padding to lay immediately within the fossa borders will create wrinkling and can lead to skin breakdown in this very fragile area.
   b. Span the fossa by having the mid point of the cast padding roll directly over the elbow flexion crease.
   c. By having the mid point of the cast padding roll directly over the elbow flexion crease, the cast padding will be slightly tented above the fossa and will not be in direct contact, thus reducing the risk of skin breakdown.
4. Because the olecranon and ulnar styloid are at risk in this splint, care should be taken to apply additional padding over these areas.

Pearls

1. A posterior elbow slab is very weak and does not provide significant immobilization.
   a. Some form of strut must be made to prevent flexion/extension.
   b. The struts can be internal to the splint or external to the splint:
      (1) Internal struts are made of plaster and applied directly to the posterior slab, providing resistance to both flexion and extension.
      (2) External struts are made of tape and applied to the splint after it is definitively secured, providing resistance to extension but not flexion.
2. Have the patient or an assistant hold the hand of the affected side by the fingertips to help with positioning and reduce pain.

Equipment

1. Cast padding: 3 inches wide
2. Plaster: 4 inches wide and 2 inches wide
3. Elastic or self-adherent bandage: 4 inches wide
4. Bucket of tepid water
5. Tape (optional): 2 inches

Basic Technique

1. Patient positioning:
   a. The patient should sit upright with his or her shoulder off the side of the bed.
   b. The elbow should be in the desired position of flexion and pronation/ supination.

2. Where to start:
   a. Proximal to the palmar flexion crease
3. Where to finish:
   a. Immediately distal to the axillary fold of the arm
4. Where to mold:
   a. Slight supracondylar mold above the elbow

Detailed Technique

1. Measure the length of the splint using plaster.
   a. Use the contralateral side.
   b. Start proximal to the palmar flexion crease.
   c. End immediately below the axillary fold.
2. Roll out the plaster.
   a. The posterior slab should be 10 to 12 layers thick and 4 inches wide.
   b. Side struts can be 8 to 10 layers thick and 2 inches wide.
3. Position the patient:
   a. Standing or sitting upright
   b. Arm freely off to the side
   c. Elbow bent to desired degree of flexion
4. Wrap the extremity in cast padding.
   a. Start at either end (Figure 13-27).
   b. Circumferentially wrap with cast padding, using a standard 50% overlap technique (see Chapter 12). Two layers of wrapping are sufficient.
   c. Carefully tear the cast padding so it conforms around the thumb interspace. Do not go past the palmar flexion crease.
   d. Span the fossa with cast padding at the antebrachial fossa (see aforementioned precautions).
   e. Tear several small strips of cast padding and apply them over the bony prominences of the olecranon and ulnar styloid to provide additional padding (Figure 13-28).

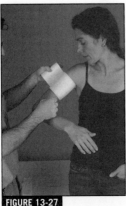

FIGURE 13-27

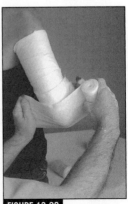

FIGURE 13-28

5. Create three cast padding cuffs (see Chapter 12):
   a. Palmar flexion crease/metacarpal heads (Figure 13-29): This cuff should form a "V" at the ulnar aspect of the hand to allow for the cascade of the digits.
   b. Thumb: This cuff should form a "V" at the base of the thumb (Figure 13-30).
   c. Proximal forearm (Figure 13-31): This cuff can be circular.
6. Prepare the plaster. Use the usual technique of wetting and laminating (see Chapter 12).
7. Apply the plaster.
   a. Apply the posterior slab first (Figure 13-32).
      (1) Position the posterior slab over the ulnar border of the forearm, around the olecranon and the posterior aspect of the arm.
      (2) Provisionally secure with cast padding at the wrist, forearm, and arm if necessary.

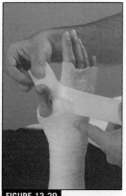

FIGURE 13-29

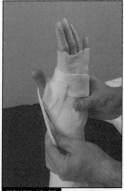

FIGURE 13-30

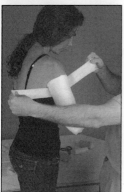

FIGURE 13-31

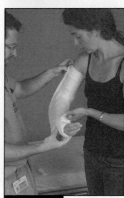

FIGURE 13-32

13

   b. Apply side struts (if not using external struts).
     (1) Start laterally at the mid arm and angle obliquely toward the forearm (Figure 13-33). Laminate the side strut to the posterior slab.
     (2) Apply the medial side strut in the same position if additional stability is needed. Laminate the side strut to the posterior slab.
8. Cover the plaster. Wrap cast padding over the top of the plaster to prevent adhesion of the plaster to the elastic or self-adherent bandage (Figure 13-34).
9. Definitively secure the splint with an elastic or self-adherent bandage (Figure 13-35).
10. Apply molding if necessary.
11. Create an external strut (if no internal struts are used) after the plaster has set (Figure 13-36). Use the figure-of-8 technique with tape.

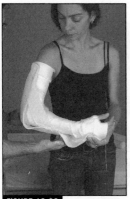

FIGURE 13-33

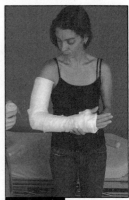

FIGURE 13-34

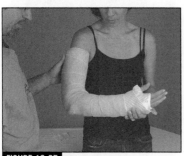

FIGURE 13-35

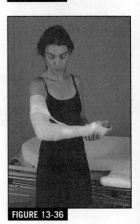

FIGURE 13-36

a. Take 2-inch silk tape and begin at the mid point of the posterior aspect of the arm (Figure 13-37)
b. Wrap around to the mid point of the anterior aspect of the arm.
c. Span the fossa obliquely.
d. Attach tape to the opposite aspect of the forearm.
e. Wrap around the dorsal forearm (Figure 13-38).
f. Span the fossa obliquely.
g. Attach tape to the lateral aspect of the arm (Figure 13-39).
h. At the intersection of the figure of 8, wrap with tape (Figure 13-40).

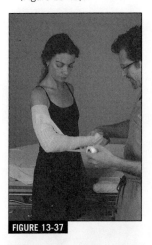

FIGURE 13-37

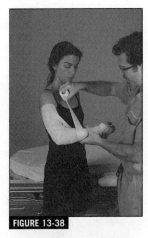

FIGURE 13-38

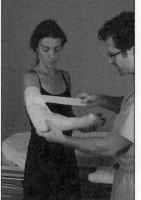

FIGURE 13-39

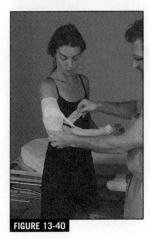

FIGURE 13-40

LONG ARM CAST

Indications for Use

1. Pediatric supracondylar humerus fractures
2. Pediatric forearm fractures
3. Pediatric unstable distal radius fractures
4. Adult distal radius fractures
5. Adult forearm fractures

Precautions

1. Do not plaster over the thenar eminence (Figure 13-41).
2. Do not extend the plaster beyond the palmar crease. The patient must be able to flex his or her metacarpophalangeal (MCP) joints to at least 70 degrees (Figure 13-42).
3. At the antecubital fossa, do not allow edges of cast padding to lay immediately within the fossa borders.
   a. Allowing edges of cast padding to lay immediately within the fossa borders will create wrinkling and can lead to skin breakdown in this very fragile area.
   b. Span the fossa by having the mid point of the cast padding roll directly over the elbow flexion crease.
   c. By having the mid point of the cast padding roll directly over the elbow flexion crease, the cast padding will be slightly tented above the fossa and will not be in direct contact, thus reducing the risk of skin breakdown.

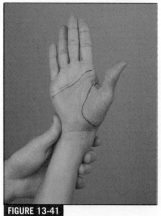

FIGURE 13-41

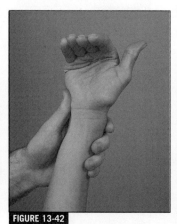

FIGURE 13-42

4. Because the olecranon and ulnar styloid are at risk in this splint, care should be taken to apply additional padding over these areas.
5. Be prepared to bivalve the cast to prevent compartment syndrome if postreduction swelling occurs.
6. Never cast an acute supracondylar fracture or floating elbow injury without bivalving.

Pearls

1. The easiest method is to create a short arm cast and then continue with the long arm portion.
2. Once you start "slinging" plaster more quickly, a long arm cast can be attempted in one step.
3. The easiest place to begin is at the wrist. The natural contour of the arm will prevent sliding.
4. It is difficult to control elbow flexion and forearm pronation when placing a long arm cast, especially in a child.
   a. To partially alleviate this difficulty, it is useful to have older children pretend they are a "drama queen" and have them place the dorsal aspect of their hand on their forehead after the short arm cast has been applied (Figure 13-43).
   b. Once the patient is in this position, the long arm portion of the cast can be completed.
   c. Parents can aid with keeping the arm at 90 degrees of elbow flexion for younger children.

Equipment

1. Stockinette: 3 to 4 inches
2. Cast padding: 3 to 4 inches
3. Plaster: 4 inches
4. Elastic or self-adherent bandage: 3 to 4 inches

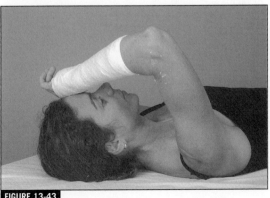

FIGURE 13-43

Basic Technique

1. Patient positioning:
   a. Supine:
      (1) Have thin patients move their body all the way to the contralateral side of the stretcher.
      (2) The patient can then rest his or her elbow on the stretcher.
   b. Upright: Use a bedside table to allow the patient to place his or her arm at a comfortable level if no reduction is required.
   c. The elbow should be bent to 90 degrees with the arm upright.
   d. The wrist position depends on the type of fracture and the location of the fracture.
      (1) Distal radius fracture:
         (a) Wrist in pronation
      (2) Fracture of both bones of the forearm:
         (a) Proximal third: wrist in supination
         (b) Middle third: wrist in neutral
         (c) Distal third: wrist in pronation
2. Where to start:
   a. Palmar flexion crease
3. Where to finish:
   a. Upper arm, below the axillary fold
4. Where to mold:
   a. Dependent on fracture
      (1) Distal radius fracture:
         (a) Same as sugar tong
      (2) Fracture of both bones of the forearm:
         (a) Interosseous mold
         (b) Ulnar-sided flat mold
5. Steps:
   a. Prepare the stockinette.
   b. Position the stockinette.
   c. Wrap the extremity in cast padding.
   d. Create three cast padding cuffs (see Chapter 12).
   e. Fold the stockinette over proximally and distally.
   f. Prepare the plaster roll in the usual fashion.
   g. Apply the plaster roll for a short arm cast.
   h. Reposition the patient.
   i. Apply the plaster roll to the elbow and arm.
   j. Split the cast, if necessary.

Detailed Technique

1. Prepare the stockinette by cutting it into two pieces:
   a. One piece for the proximal portion at the arm
   b. One piece for the distal portion at the hand
2. Position the stockinette:
   a. Place one stockinette over the upper arm.
   b. Cut a thumb hole in the mid portion of the other stockinette and fit this piece over the hand (**Figure 13-44**).
   c. The stockinette should extend to the proximal interphalangeal (PIP) joints.
3. Wrap the extremity in cast padding.
   a. Start at the wrist and circumferentially wrap distally (**Figure 13-45**).
      (1) Use a standard 50% overlap technique (see Chapter 12).
      (2) Two layers of padding are sufficient.

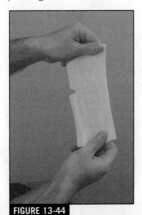

FIGURE 13-44

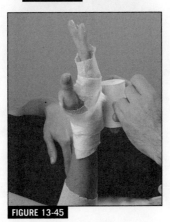

FIGURE 13-45

13

    b. Carefully tear the cast padding so as to conform around the thumb
       interspace (Figure 13-46). Do not go past the palmar flexion crease.
    c. Once the hand has been adequately padded, continue wrapping
       proximally to the proximal forearm (Figure 13-47).
    d. Span the fossa with cast padding at the antebrachial fossa
       (Figure 13-48) (see aforementioned precautions).
    e. Continue proximally to area just below axillary fold (Figure 13-49).
4. Create three cast padding cuffs (see Chapter 12).
    a. Palmar flexion crease/metacarpal heads (see Figure 13-29): This
       cuff should form a "V" at the ulnar aspect of the hand to allow for the
       cascade of the digits.

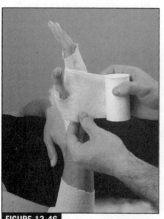

FIGURE 13-46

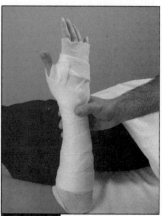

FIGURE 13-47

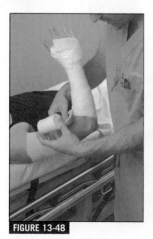

FIGURE 13-48

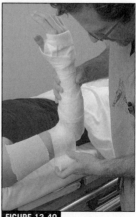

FIGURE 13-49

    b. Thumb: Again, form a "V" at the base of the thumb (see Figure 13-30).

    c. Proximal arm (Figure 13-50): This cuff can be circular.

5. Fold the stockinette over proximally and distally. Ensure that MCP motion is completely preserved.

6. Prepare the plaster roll in the usual fashion (see Chapter 12).

7. Apply the plaster roll for a short arm cast.

    a. Start at the wrist and work distally.

    b. Use a twisting (Figure 13-51) or pinching (Figure 13-52) motion to get through the thumb interspace. Twist the plaster roll 360 degrees in the interspace.

    c. Roll two more times around the hand and through the thumb interspace.

    d. Continue the plaster proximally (Figure 13-53). Use the standard technique of laminating while rolling (see Chapter 12).

    e. Ensure that at least 3 to 5 layers of plaster are applied.

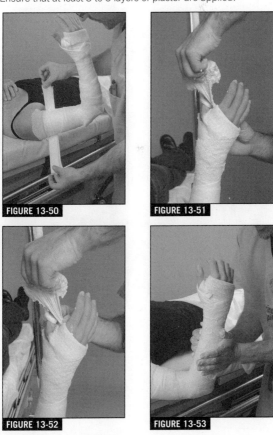

FIGURE 13-50

FIGURE 13-51

FIGURE 13-52

FIGURE 13-53

13

8. Reposition the patient if using the "drama queen" technique.
   a. The patient should be supine.
   b. The hand is on the forehead with the elbow flexed to 90 degrees.
9. Apply a plaster roll to the elbow and arm. Be vigilant about avoiding patient movement when applying this portion of the cast.
10. Apply a mold, if desired. For a fracture of both bones of the forearm:
    a. An interosseous mold should be made over the forearm by compressing the anterior and posterior surfaces to make the cast more oval and less cylindrical (Figure 13-54).
    b. A straight ulnar border also is applied to prevent the fracture from falling to varus.
       (1) A straight ulnar border can be applied at the same time as the interosseous mold (Figure 13-55).

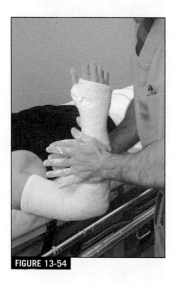

FIGURE 13-54

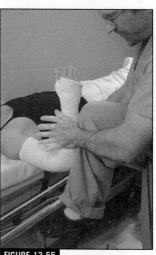

FIGURE 13-55

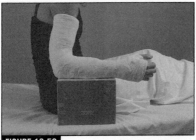

FIGURE 13-56

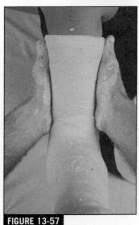

FIGURE 13-57

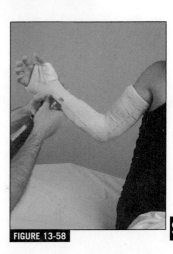

FIGURE 13-58

13

  (2) Alternatively, after applying an interosseous mold, place the
      ulnar side of the cast on a hard flat surface to make sure it is flat
      (Figure 13-56).
  c. A supracondylar humerus mold also can be applied if desired
     (Figure 13-57).
11. Split the cast if necessary (Figure 13-58).

SUGAR-TONG SPLINT

Indications for Use

Distal radius fractures

Precautions

1. It is crucial that the splint be neither too long nor too short.
   a. If the splint is too long and extends beyond the metacarpal heads,
      finger flexion is significantly impaired and permanent finger stiffness
      or contractures may ensue.
   b. If the splint is too short, the reduction will not hold.

2. Do not immobilize the thumb. This error is extremely common. Remember, the thumb must be able to oppose and thus, unlike the fingers, its range of motion begins at the basal joint (carpometacarpal joint).
3. Do not mold the splint in such a fashion that the wrist is flexed beyond 10 to 15 degrees; otherwise acute carpal tunnel syndrome may occur!

Pearls

1. The normal cascade of the fingers slopes downward from the index to the little finger.
   a. A 30-degree cut can be made in one end of the plaster slab to incorporate this cascade.
   b. A curvilinear cut can be made to free the thenar eminence about the thumb (Figures 13-59 and 13-60).
2. Before measuring the splint, it may be useful to perform a hematoma block, thus allowing the block to become effective while the splint is being measured.
3. It is better to measure the splint long rather than short. The splint can always be trimmed or folded over during application if it is too long, but a new splint will need to be made if it is too short.
4. The cast padding may be measured 1 to 2 inches long on the volar aspect so that it may be folded over the end of the plaster splint, thus providing a comfortable and safe edge to the splint.
5. The sugar-tong splint has a tendency to become very bulky at the elbow.

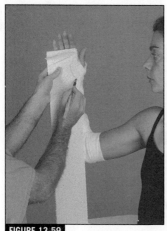

FIGURE 13-59

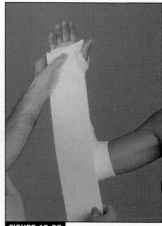

FIGURE 13-60

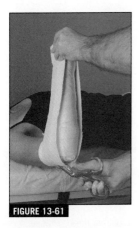

FIGURE 13-61

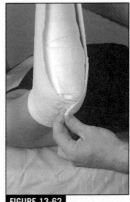

FIGURE 13-62

a. To prevent bulkiness at the elbow, a small cut is made in the plaster at the elbow once it has been applied and provisionally fixed (Figure 13-61).
b. The free ends are folded over one another to conform to the curvature of the flexed elbow (Figure 13-62).

Equipment

1. Stockinette: 3 inches
2. Cast padding: 3 to 4 inches
3. Plaster: 3 to 4 inches
4. Elastic or self-adherent bandage: 3 to 4 inches
5. Portable radiograph machine (optional)

Basic Technique

1. Patient positioning:
   a. The patient is either supine on the stretcher with the entire shoulder girdle off the side or the patient is sitting or standing.
   b. The elbow is bent at 90 degrees.
   c. The splint may be applied while the patient is in traction (see Chapter 10).
2. Where to start:
   a. Volar (palmar) aspect, immediately below the palmar crease
3. Where to finish:
   a. Dorsal aspect, immediately below the metacarpal heads
4. Where to mold (3-point mold):
   a. For a dorsally angulated distal radius fracture:
      (1) Dorsal aspect of the carpus
      (2) Volar forearm immediately proximal to the wrist crease
      (3) Dorsal aspect of the forearm
   b. For a volarly angulated distal radius fracture:
      (1) Volar aspect of the carpus
      (2) Dorsal forearm immediately proximal to the wrist crease
      (3) Volar aspect of the forearm

5. Steps:
   a. Measure the length of the splint using plaster.
   b. Roll out the plaster.
   c. Roll out the cast padding.
   d. Position the patient.
   e. Set traction, if necessary.
   f. Obtain traction views, if necessary.
   g. Perform a reduction maneuver, if necessary.
   h. Prepare plaster in the usual fashion.
   i. Apply a splint.
   j. Definitively secure the splint with an elastic bandage.
   k. Perform a three-point mold.

Detailed Technique

1. Measure the length of the splint using plaster (Figure 13-63).
   a. Use the contralateral side.
   b. Start the volar (palmar) aspect at the palmar flexion crease.
   c. Wrap around the elbow and finish at the metacarpal heads.
2. Roll out the plaster. The plaster slab should be 10 sheets thick.
3. Roll out the cast padding. Use the usual technique that will allow the padding to be folded over (see Chapter 12).
4. Position the patient:
   a. The patient should be supine on the stretcher with the shoulder girdle entirely off the side.
   b. Prepare finger traps if using traction (see Chapter 10).
   c. Abduct the shoulder to 90 degrees and flex the elbow to 90 degrees to create a 90-90 position.
5. Set traction, if necessary.
6. Obtain traction views, if necessary (this step may be performed following the reduction maneuver, as desired).
7. Perform a reduction maneuver, if necessary (see Chapter 10).

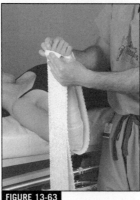

FIGURE 13-63

8. Prepare plaster in the usual fashion, with wetting and laminating, followed by placement in cast padding (see Chapter 12).
9. Apply a splint.
   a. Begin at the volar aspect. Do not go past the palmar crease.
   b. Wrap the splint around the elbow.
   c. Provisionally secure the splint at the wrist with cast padding (Figure 13-64).
   d. Ensure that the edges of the splint are at the correct length.
      (1) If the edges are too long, fold them over.
      (2) If the edges are too short, the splint will need to be remade.
   e. Cut a slit in the splint at the elbow to prevent bulk (see Figure 13-61). Fold the edges over one another (see Figure 13-62).
10. Definitively secure the splint with elastic or a self-adherent bandage.
    a. Start at the elbow.
    b. Ensure that the elastic or self-adherent bandage has only minimal contact with the skin.
    c. Wrap the elastic or self-adherent bandage distally. A hole can be cut out for the thumb, if desired (Figure 13-65).
    d. Secure the end with silk tape if needed (Figure 13-66).
11. Perform a three-point mold, if desired.

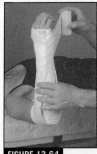

FIGURE 13-64

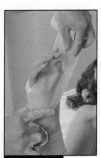

FIGURE 13-65

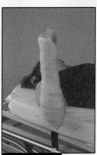

FIGURE 13-66

THUMB SPICA SPLINT

Indications for Use

1. Scaphoid fractures
2. Thumb metacarpal fractures
3. Thumb carpometacarpal dislocations

Precautions

Be careful not to create a mold that is too dramatic, because the indentation in the plaster can lead to skin necrosis and pressure sores.

Pearls

1. The application of cast padding is the most important aspect of this splint.
2. Careful attention should be paid to the area around the thumb to avoid bunching and wrinkles.

Equipment

1. Stockinette: 3 inches
2. Cast padding: 3 inches
3. Plaster: 4 inches
4. Elastic or self-adherent bandage: 3 inches

Basic Technique

1. Patient positioning:
   a. The elbow is bent to 90 degrees with the arm upright.
   b. Supine:
      (1) Have patients who are thin move their body all the way to the contralateral side of the stretcher.
      (2) The patient can then rest his or her elbow on the stretcher.
   c. Upright:
      (1) Use a bedside table to allow the patient to place his or her arm at a comfortable level.
2. Where to start:
   a. Distal to the thumb interphalangeal (IP) joint for thumb fractures
   b. Just proximal to the IP joint for scaphoid fractures
3. Where to finish:
   a. Mid to proximal forearm
4. Where to mold:
   a. The thumb should be abducted 30 degrees away from the hand, in its neutral position.

5. Steps:
   a. Measure the length of the splint using plaster.
   b. Roll out the plaster.
   c. Wrap the extremity in cast padding.
   d. Create three cast padding cuffs.
   e. Prepare the plaster.
   f. Apply the plaster.
   g. Cover the plaster.
   h. Definitively secure the splint with an elastic or self-adherent bandage.

Detailed Technique

1. Measure the length of the splint using plaster (Figure 13-67). Start at the thumb and go to the mid to proximal forearm.
2. Roll out the plaster. The plaster slab should be 10 sheets thick.
3. Wrap the extremity in cast padding
   a. Start at the wrist and circumferentially wrap distally to the hand (Figure 13-68).
      (1) Use a standard 50% overlap technique (see Chapter 12).
      (2) Two layers of wrapping are sufficient.
   b. Carefully tear the cast padding so as to conform around the thumb interspace (Figure 13-69). Do not go past the palmar flexion crease.

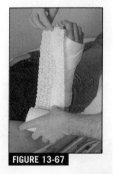

FIGURE 13-67

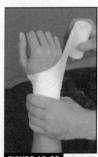

FIGURE 13-68

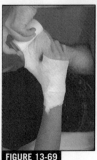

FIGURE 13-69

c. Once the hand has been adequately padded, continue wrapping proximally to the mid forearm (Figure 13-70).
4. Create three cast padding cuffs (see Chapter 12):
   a. Palmar flexion crease/metacarpal heads: The cuff should form a "V" at the ulnar aspect of the hand to allow for the cascade of the digits (Figures 13-71 and 13-72).

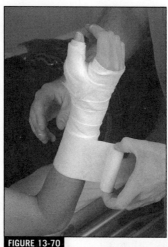

FIGURE 13-70

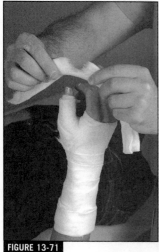

FIGURE 13-71

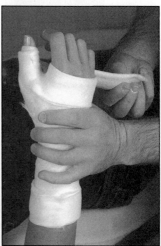

FIGURE 13-72

    b. Thumb: Padding cuff at the tip of the thumb (Figure 13-73).
    c. Proximal forearm: This cuff can be circular (Figure 13-74).
5. Prepare the plaster. Employ the usual technique of wetting and laminating (see Chapter 12).
6. Apply the plaster:
    a. Position the plaster on the radial border of the thumb and forearm (Figure 13-75).
    b. Provisionally secure the plaster at the wrist with cast padding (Figure 13-76).
7. Cover the plaster. Place strips of cast padding over the top of the plaster to protect the elastic bandage.

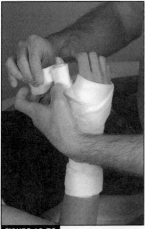

FIGURE 13-73

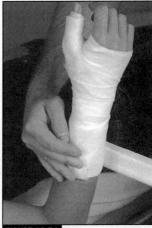

FIGURE 13-74

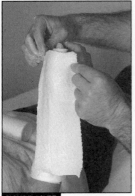

FIGURE 13-75

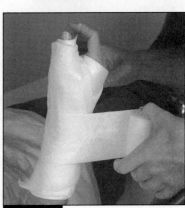

FIGURE 13-76

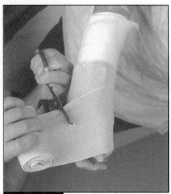

FIGURE 13-77

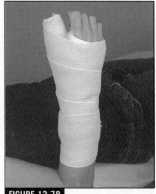

FIGURE 13-78

8. Definitively secure the plaster with an elastic bandage:
   a. Begin at the thumb and work distally.
   b. An opening for the thumb web space can be cut into the elastic or self-adherent bandage (Figure 13-77).
   c. Work distally to the mid forearm (Figure 13-78).
   d. Secure the end with silk tape.

SHORT ARM CAST

Indications for Use

1. Distal radius fracture (nonacute)
2. Nonscaphoid carpal fractures
3. Distal ulna fracture

Precautions

1. Do not plaster over the thenar eminence (see Figure 13-41).
2. Do not extend the plaster beyond the palmar crease. The patient must be able to flex his or her MCPs to 90 degrees (see Figure 13-42).
3. Bony prominences, such as the ulnar styloid, must be well padded. Additional strips of padding may be applied over these potential pressure points.

Pearls

The easiest place to begin is at the wrist. The natural contour of the arm will prevent sliding.

Equipment

1. Stockinette: 3 inches
2. Cast padding: 3 inches
3. Plaster: 3 inches
4. Elastic or self-adherent bandage: 3 inches

Basic Technique

1. Patient positioning:
   a. The elbow should be bent to 90 degrees with the arm upright.
   b. Supine:
      (1) Have thin patients move their body all the way to the contralateral side of the stretcher.
      (2) The patient can then rest his or her elbow on the stretcher.
   c. Upright: Use a bedside table to allow the patient to place his or her arm at a comfortable level.
2. Where to start:
   a. Palmar flexion crease
3. Where to finish:
   a. Mid forearm
4. Where to mold (three-point mold):
   a. For a dorsally angulated or displaced distal radius fracture:
      (1) Dorsal aspect of carpus
      (2) Volar distal forearm
      (3) Dorsal aspect of the mid forearm
   b. For a volarly angulated or displaced distal radius fracture:
      (1) Volar aspect of the carpus
      (2) Dorsal distal forearm immediately proximal to the wrist crease
      (3) Volar aspect of the mid forearm
5. Steps:
   a. Prepare a stockinette.
   b. Position the stockinette.
   c. Wrap the extremity in cast padding.
   d. Create three cast padding cuffs.
   e. Fold the stockinette over both proximally and distally.
   f. Prepare the plaster roll in the usual fashion.
   g. Apply the plaster roll.
   h. Split the cast, if necessary.

Detailed Technique

1. Prepare a stockinette by cutting it into two pieces:
   a. One piece for the proximal portion at the elbow
   b. One piece for the distal portion at the hand

2. Position the stockinette:
   a. Place one stockinette over the elbow with equal lengths on either side.
   b. Cut a thumb hole in the mid portion of the other stockinette and fit this portion over the hand (Figure 13-79).
   c. The stockinette should extend to the PIP joints.
3. Wrap the extremity in cast padding.
   a. Start at the wrist and circumferentially wrap distally (Figure 13-80).
      (1) Use a standard 50% overlap technique (see Chapter 12).
      (2) Two layers of padding are sufficient.

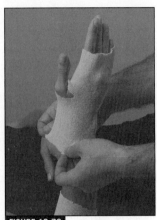

FIGURE 13-79

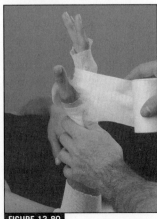

FIGURE 13-80

   b. Carefully tear the cast padding so as to conform around the thumb interspace. Do not go past the palmar flexion crease.

   c. Once the hand has been adequately padded, continue wrapping proximally to the proximal forearm (Figure 13-81).

4. Create three cast padding cuffs (see Chapter 12):

   a. Palmar flexion crease/metacarpal heads (see Figure 13-29): This cuff should form a "V" at the ulnar aspect of the hand to allow for the cascade of the digits (Figure 13-82).

   b. Thumb: Again, form a "V" at the base of the thumb (see Figure 13-30).

   c. Proximal forearm (Figure 13-83): This cuff can be circular.

5. Fold the stockinette over both proximally and distally. Ensure that MCP motion is completely preserved (Figure 13-84).

6. Prepare the plaster roll in the usual fashion (see Chapter 12).

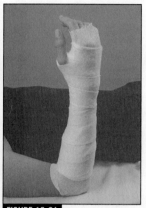
FIGURE 13-81

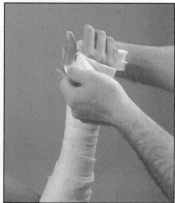
FIGURE 13-82

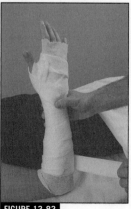
FIGURE 13-83

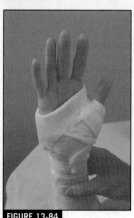
FIGURE 13-84

13

7. Apply the plaster roll.
   a. Start at the wrist and work distally (Figure 13-85).
   b. Use a twisting motion to get through the thumb interspace.
      (1) Twist the plaster roll 360 degrees in the interspace (Figure 13-86).
      (2) Alternatively, if using fiberglass, the fiberglass can be cut to conform to the thumb interspace (Figure 13-87).
   c. Roll two more times around the hand and through the thumb interspace. Do not go past the palmar flexion crease (Figure 13-88).

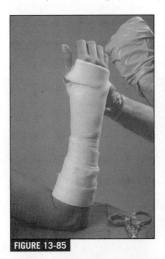
FIGURE 13-85

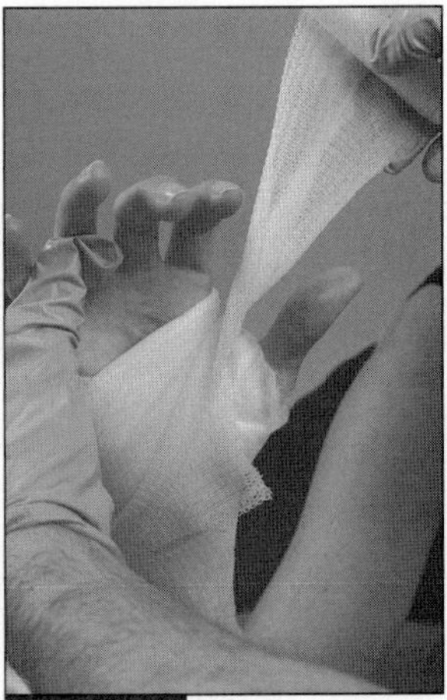

FIGURE 13-86

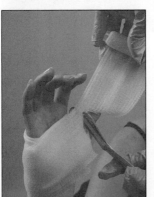
FIGURE 13-87

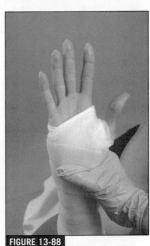
FIGURE 13-88

d. Continue the plaster proximally (Figure 13-89). Use the standard technique of laminating while rolling (see Chapter 12).
e. Ensure that at least three to five layers of plaster are applied.
8. Split the cast, if necessary.

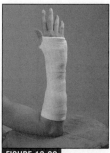

FIGURE 13-89

THUMB SPICA CAST

Indications for Use

Scaphoid fracture (nonacute)

Precautions

1. Do not extend the plaster beyond the palmar crease. The patient must be able to flex his or her MCP joints to 90 degrees.
2. Bony prominences, such as the ulnar styloid, must be well padded. Additional strips of padding may be applied over these potential pressure points.

Pearls

1. The easiest place to begin is at the wrist. The natural contour of the arm will prevent sliding.
2. For proximal phalangeal fractures or MCP joint dislocations, a hand-based thumb spica cast can be used (Figure 13-90).
   a. A hand-based thumb spica cast begins just distal to the wrist crease and extends to cover the entire thumb.
   b. A hand-based thumb spica cast allows wrist motion.

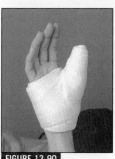

FIGURE 13-90

Equipment

1. Stockinette: 3 inches
2. Cast padding: 3 inches
3. Plaster: 3 inches
4. Elastic or self-adherent bandage: 3 inches

Basic Technique

1. Patient positioning:
   a. The elbow should be bent to 90 degrees with the arm upright.
   b. Supine:
      (1) Have thin patients move their body all the way to the contralateral side of the stretcher.
      (2) The patient can then rest his or her elbow on the stretcher.
   c. Upright: Use a bedside table to allow the patient to place his or her arm at a comfortable level.
2. Where to start:
   a. Thumb:
      (1) Distal to the interphalangeal (IP) joint for injuries at or distal to the metaphalangeal (MP) joint
      (2) Proximal to IP joint for injuries proximal to MP joint
   b. Hand:
      (1) Proximal to the distal palmar crease
3. Where to finish:
   a. Upper forearm
4. Where to mold:
   a. Interosseous mold
5. Steps:
   a. Prepare a stockinette.
   b. Position the stockinette.
   c. Wrap the extremity in cast padding.
   d. Create three cast padding cuffs.
   e. Fold the stockinette over both proximally and distally.
   f. Prepare the plaster roll in the usual fashion.
   g. Apply the plaster roll.
   h. Split the cast if necessary.

Detailed Technique

1. Prepare the stockinette by cutting it in two pieces:
   a. One piece is for the proximal portion at the elbow
   b. One piece is for the distal portion at the hand

2. Position the stockinette (Figure 13-91).
   a. Place one stockinette over the elbow with equal lengths on either side.
   b. Cut a thumb hole in the mid portion of the other stockinette and fit this portion over the hand (Figure 13-92).
   c. The stockinette should extend to the PIP joints.
3. Wrap the extremity in cast padding.
   a. Start at the wrist and circumferentially wrap distally (Figure 13-93).
      (1) Use a standard 50% overlap technique (see Chapter 12).
      (2) Two layers of padding are sufficient.
   b. Carefully tear the cast padding so as to conform around the thumb interspace (Figure 13-94). Do not go past the palmar flexion crease.

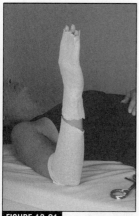

FIGURE 13-91

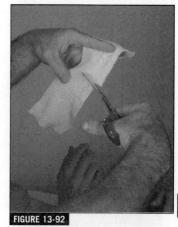

FIGURE 13-92

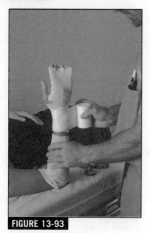

FIGURE 13-93

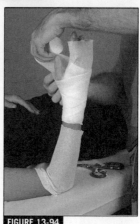

FIGURE 13-94

13

c. Tear several strips of cast padding to pad the thumb.
d. Once the hand has been adequately padded, continue wrapping proximally to the proximal forearm.
4. Create three cast padding cuffs (see Chapter 12):
   a. Palmar flexion crease/metacarpal heads: This cuff should form a "V" at the ulnar aspect of the hand to allow for the cascade of the digits (Figure 13-95).
   b. Thumb: This cuff can be circular distal to the IP joint (Figure 13-96).
   c. Proximal forearm (Figure 13-97): This cuff can be circular.
5. Fold the stockinette over both proximally and distally (Figure 13-98). Ensure that MP joint motion is completely preserved.
6. Prepare the plaster roll in the usual fashion (see Chapter 12).

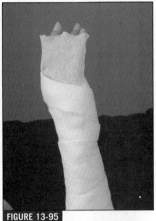

FIGURE 13-95

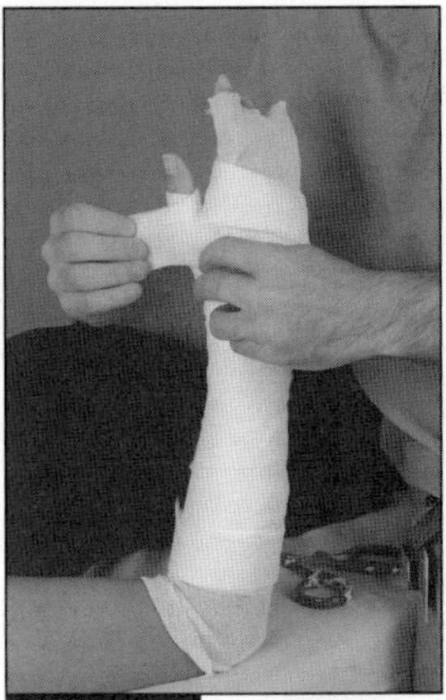

FIGURE 13-96

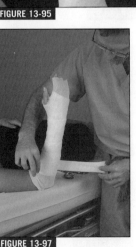

FIGURE 13-97

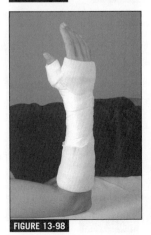

FIGURE 13-98

7. Apply the plaster roll.
   a. Start at the wrist and work distally.
   b. Use a twisting or pinching motion to get through the thumb
      interspace.
      (1) Twist the plaster roll 360 degrees in the interspace (Figure 13-99).
      (2) Pinch the roll to narrow it at the web space (Figure 13-100).
   c. Roll two more times around the hand and through the thumb interspace.
   d. Roll around the thumb, being careful not to extend beyond the cast
      padding.
   e. Continue the plaster proximally (Figures 13-101 and 13-102).
      (1) Use the standard technique of laminating while rolling
          (Chapter 12).
   f. Ensure that at least three to five layers of plaster are applied.

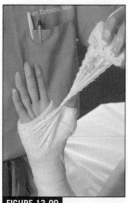

FIGURE 13-99

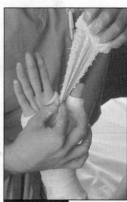

FIGURE 13-100

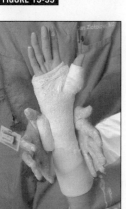

FIGURE 13-101

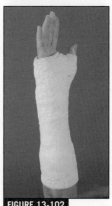

FIGURE 13-102

13

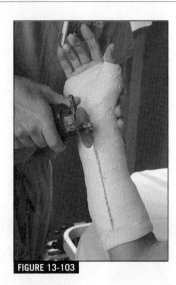

FIGURE 13-103

8. Mold the cast, if desired. An interosseous mold over the forearm should be made by compressing the anterior and posterior surfaces to make the cast more oval and less cylindrical.
9. Split the cast, if necessary (Figure 13-103).

ULNAR GUTTER SPLINT

Overview

1. Two techniques are described for creation of an ulnar gutter splint:
   a. One plaster
   b. Two-plaster dorsal-ulnar
2. Either of these techniques will ensure a strong ulnar gutter splint.
   a. The two-plaster dorsal-ulnar splint is typically easiest for the novice to apply.
   b. The one-plaster ulnar gutter splint is an alternative technique that some expert individuals find easiest to apply.

Indications for Use

1. Ring and little finger metacarpal and proximal phalangeal fractures
2. Most commonly applied for a little finger metacarpal neck fracture, better known as a "boxer's fracture"

Precautions

1. Immobilization of the digits in the intrinsic plus position is key to preventing complications (see Chapter 12).
2. Cast padding should be placed between the immobilized digits to prevent maceration of the skin.

Pearls

1. Having the patient positioned so that his or her elbow may rest on a table (or another hard surface) greatly simplifies the application of this splint.
2. Measure the plaster long, because this splint is difficult to measure prior to application.
3. For injuries of the MP joint or the proximal phalanx, a hand-based splint can be used.

Technique 1: One Plaster

Equipment

1. Cast padding: 3 inches
2. Plaster: 4 inches
3. Elastic or self-adherent bandage: 3 inches

Basic Technique

1. Patient positioning:
   a. The elbow is bent to 90 degrees with the arm upright.
   b. Supine:
      (1) Have thin patients move their body all the way to the contralateral side of the stretcher.
      (2) The patient can then rest his or her elbow on the stretcher.
   c. Upright: Use a bedside table to allow the patient to place his or her arm at a comfortable level.
2. Where to start:
   a. For a metacarpal fracture: PIP joint
   b. For a phalangeal fracture: fingertip
3. Where to finish:
   a. For a metacarpal fracture: proximal third of the forearm
   b. For a phalangeal fracture: just distal to the wrist
4. Where to mold:
   a. Dorsum over metacarpal
   b. Dorsum over phalanges; the volar mold will largely occur by virtue of bending
5. Steps:
   a. Measure the length of the splint using plaster.
   b. Wrap the ring and little fingers in cast padding.
   c. Roll out the plaster.
   d. Roll out the cast padding.
   e. Prepare the plaster.
   f. Apply the splint.
   g. Mold the splint.
   h. Definitively secure the splint with an elastic bandage.
   i. Perform a reduction maneuver, if necessary.

13

Detailed Technique

1. Measure the length of the splint (Figure 13-104).
   a. Use the contralateral side.
   b. Measure from the PIP to the proximal third of the forearm along the ulnar aspect of the limb.
2. Wrap the extremity in cast padding.
   a. Start at the mid forearm and circumferentially wrap distally (Figure 13-105).
      (1) Use a standard 50% overlap technique (see Chapter 12).
      (2) Two layers of padding are sufficient.
   b. Carefully tear the cast padding so as to conform around the thumb interspace (Figure 13-106). Do not go past the palmar flexion crease.
   c. Wrap the ring and little fingers in cast padding.
      (1) Begin by placing a small piece of folded cast padding between the ring and little fingers (Figure 13-107) to prevent maceration between the digits.

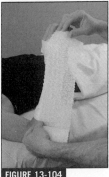

FIGURE 13-104

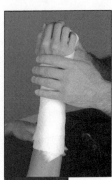

FIGURE 13-105

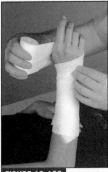

FIGURE 13-106

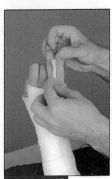

FIGURE 13-107

(2) Create a cast padding cuff (Figure 13-108). Wrap around the proximal portion of ring and little fingers (Figure 13-109).
(3) Using 2-inch cast padding, apply two layers over the dorsum of the ring and little fingers that extends to the PIP joint or fingertip (Figure 13-110).
(4) Create a cast padding cuff (Figure 13-111):

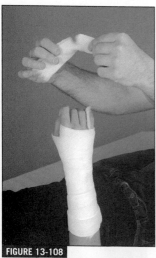

FIGURE 13-108

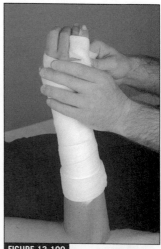

FIGURE 13-109

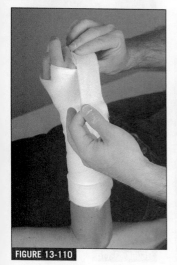

FIGURE 13-110

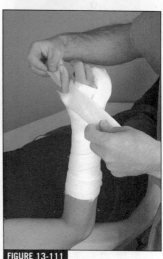

FIGURE 13-111

(a) Palmar flexion crease/metacarpal heads **(Figure 13-112)**: This cuff should form a "V" at the ulnar aspect of the hand to allow for the cascade of the digits.

(5) Create a cast padding cuff **(Figure 13-113)**. Wrap around the distal portion of the ring and little fingers **(Figure 13-114)**.

(6) The digits should be well-padded at this point, with the index and long fingers completely free **(Figure 13-115)**. (If desired, an additional cuff can be placed around the thumb, as illustrated.)

3. Roll out the plaster. The plaster slab should be 10 sheets thick.
4. Prepare the plaster. Employ the usual technique of wetting and laminating (see Chapter 12).

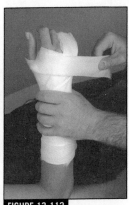

FIGURE 13-112

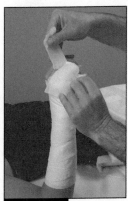

FIGURE 13-113

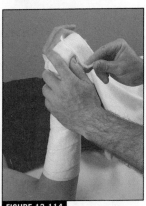

FIGURE 13-114

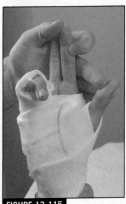

FIGURE 13-115

5. Apply the splint.
   a. Start by applying the splint to the dorsal side of the forearm (Figure 13-116). Ensure appropriate placement distally.
   b. Wrap around the ulnar digits.
   c. Wrap around the forearm (Figure 13-117).
   d. Provisionally secure with cast padding (Figure 13-118).
6. Mold the splint (Figure 13-119).
   a. Place one hand on the volar aspect of the palm.
   b. With the other hand, mold the dorsal aspect of the plaster to 90 degrees.

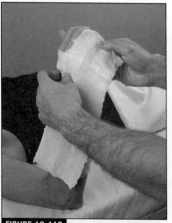

FIGURE 13-116

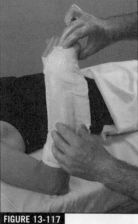

FIGURE 13-117

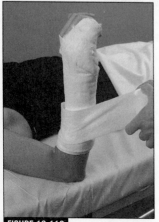

FIGURE 13-118

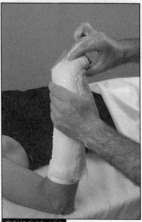

FIGURE 13-119

13

7. Perform a reduction maneuver if necessary.
8. Mold the splint (Figure 13-120).
   a. Place one hand on the wrist with the thumb pressing on the dorsum of the metacarpal shaft.
   b. With the other hand, cup the ulnar digits to allow axial compression and positioning of the MP joint at 90 degrees.
9. Definitively secure the splint with an elastic or self-adherent bandage.
   a. Begin at the wrist and work distally (Figure 13-121).
   b. Secure the end with silk tape.

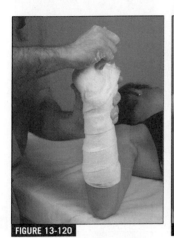

FIGURE 13-120

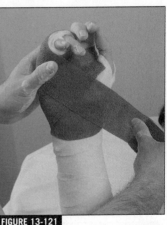

FIGURE 13-121

Technique 2: Two-Plaster, Dorsal-Ulnar Placement Modification

Equipment

1. Cast padding: 2 inches
2. Plaster: 2 inches
3. Elastic or self-adherent bandage: 3 inches

Basic Technique

1. The extremity is positioned and padded as in technique 1.
2. Two overlapping plaster slabs are used instead of one.

Detailed Technique

1. Measure the length of the splint.
   a. Use the contralateral side.
   b. Take two measurements:
      (1) Measure one slab along the dorsum of the hand/forearm.
      (2) Measure another slab perpendicular to the first, starting at the dorsum of the hand and down the ulnar side of the hand/forearm.
2. Roll out the plaster.
   a. Two plaster slabs should be created, based on the aforementioned measurement.
   b. Each plaster slab should be 10 sheets thick.
3. Wrap the extremity in cast padding (see technique 1).
4. Prepare the plaster. Employ the usual technique of wetting and laminating (see Chapter 12).
5. Apply the plaster.
   a. Start by applying one slab to the dorsal side of the fingers and extend proximally down the ulnar border of the forearm (Figure 13-122). Provisionally secure it with cast padding at the fingers and wrist.
   b. Place a second slab along the dorsum of the fingers and forearm (Figure 13-123). Provisionally secure it with cast padding at the wrist and fingers.

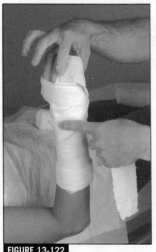

FIGURE 13-122

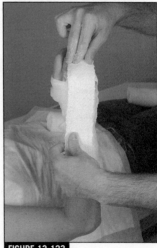

FIGURE 13-123

   c. The proximal part of the ulnar strip can be moved in a volar direction to aid with maintaining the position of the splint (Figure 13-124).

6. Cover the plaster: Place cast padding over the top of the plaster to prevent the covering bandage from sticking to the plaster (Figure 13-125).

7. Mold the splint (see technique 1).

8. Perform a reduction maneuver, if necessary.

9. Definitively secure the splint with an elastic or self-adherent bandage (Figure 13-126).

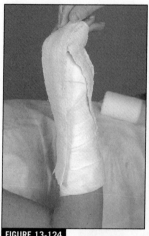

FIGURE 13-124

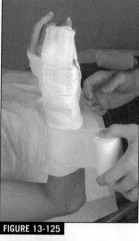

FIGURE 13-125

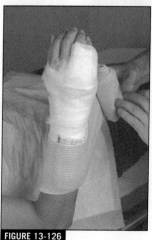

FIGURE 13-126

a. The bandage can be cut (Figure 13-127) to minimize bulk between the long and ring digits (Figure 13-128).
b. The bandage can be cut (Figure 13-129) to accommodate the thumb (Figure 13-130).
c. Secure the end with silk tape.

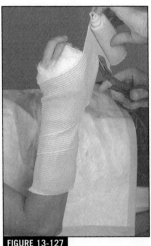

FIGURE 13-127

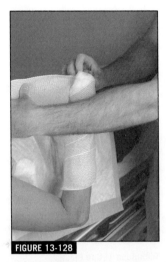

FIGURE 13-128

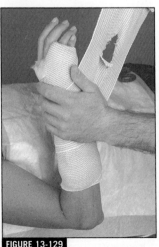

FIGURE 13-129

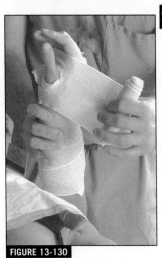

FIGURE 13-130

RADIAL GUTTER SPLINT

Overview

1. The radial gutter splint is similar to an ulnar gutter splint except that it immobilizes the index and long finger.
2. Because of the thumb, two techniques can be used.
   a. A two-plaster dorsal-volar technique can be used.
   b. A single slab with a fenestration for the thumb also can be used.

Indications for Use

Index and long finger metacarpal and proximal phalangeal fractures

Precautions

1. Immobilization of the digits in the intrinsic plus position is key to preventing complications (see Chapter 12).
2. Cast padding should be placed between the immobilized digits to prevent maceration of the skin.
3. When placing the elastic bandage, do not wrap over the thenar eminence.

Pearls

1. Having the patient positioned so that his or her elbow may rest on a table (or other hard surface) greatly simplifies the application of this splint.
2. Measure the plaster long, because this splint is difficult to measure prior to application.
3. For injuries of the MP joint or the proximal phalanx, a hand-based splint can be used.

Technique 1: One Plaster

Equipment

1. Cast padding: 3 inches
2. Plaster: 4 inches
3. Elastic or self-adherent bandage: 3 inches

Basic Technique

1. Patient positioning:
   a. The elbow is bent to 90 degrees with the arm upright.
   b. Supine:
      (1) Have patients who are thin move their body all the way to the contralateral side of the stretcher.
      (2) The patient can then rest his or her elbow on the stretcher.
   c. Upright: Use a bedside table to allow the patient to place his or her arm at a comfortable level.
2. Where to start:
   a. For a metacarpal fracture: PIP joint
   b. For a phalangeal fracture: fingertip
3. Where to finish:
   a. For a metacarpal fracture: proximal third of the forearm
   b. For a phalangeal fracture: just distal to the wrist

4. Where to mold:
   a. Dorsum over metacarpal
   b. Dorsum over phalanges; the volar mold will largely occur by virtue of bending
5. Steps:
   a. Measure the length of the splint using plaster.
   b. Wrap the ring and little fingers in cast padding.
   c. Roll out the plaster.
   d. Roll out the cast padding.
   e. Prepare the plaster.
   f. Apply the splint.
   g. Mold the splint.
   h. Definitively secure the splint with an elastic bandage.
   i. Perform a reduction maneuver, if necessary.

Detailed Technique

1. Measure the length of the splint.
   a. Use the contralateral side.
   b. Measure from the DIP to the proximal third of the forearm along the ulnar aspect of the limb.
2. Wrap the extremity in cast padding.
   a. Start at the mid forearm and circumferentially wrap distally.
      (1) Use a standard 50% overlap technique (see Chapter 12).
      (2) Two layers of padding are sufficient.
   b. Carefully tear the cast padding so as to conform around the thumb interspace. Do not go past the palmar flexion crease.
   c. Wrap the index and long fingers in cast padding (Figure 13-131).
      (1) Begin by placing a small piece of folded cast padding between the long and index fingers (Figure 13-132) to prevent maceration between the digits.

13

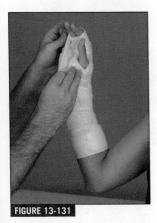

FIGURE 13-131

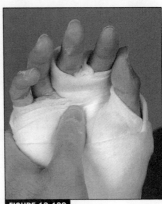

FIGURE 13-132

(2) Create a cast padding cuff. Wrap it around the proximal portion of the index and long fingers.

(3) Using 2-inch cast padding, apply two layers over the dorsum of the index and long fingers.

(4) Create a cast padding cuff.

    (a) Palmar flexion crease/metacarpal heads: This cuff should form a "V" at the ulnar aspect of the hand to allow for the cascade of the digits.

(5) Create a cast padding cuff. Wrap it around the distal portion of the index and long fingers.

(6) The digits should be well-padded at this point, with the ring and small fingers completely free (**Figure 13-133**). (If desired, an additional cuff can be placed around the thumb, as illustrated.)

3. Roll out the plaster.

    a. The plaster slab should be 10 sheets thick.

    b. Fold and cut a hole to accommodate the thumb (**Figure 13-134**).

4. Prepare the plaster. Employ the usual technique of wetting and laminating (see Chapter 12).

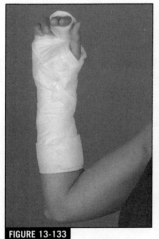

FIGURE 13-133

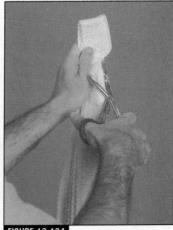

FIGURE 13-134

5. Apply the plaster.
   a. Start by applying the plaster to the radial side of the forearm (Figure 13-135). Ensure appropriate placement distally.
   b. Wrap around digits and secure with cast padding (Figure 13-136).
6. Perform a reduction maneuver, if necessary.
7. Mold the splint (Figure 13-137):
   a. Place one hand on the wrist with thumb pressing on the dorsum of the metacarpal shaft.
   b. With the other hand, cup the radial digits to allow axial compression and positioning of the MP joint at 90 degrees.

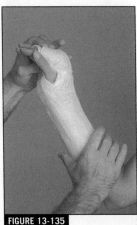

FIGURE 13-135

13

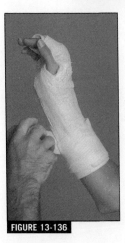

FIGURE 13-136

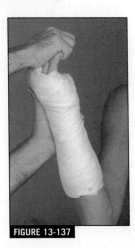

FIGURE 13-137

8. Definitively secure the splint with an elastic or self-adherent bandage.
   a. Begin at the wrist and work distally (Figure 13-138).
   b. Secure the end with silk tape.

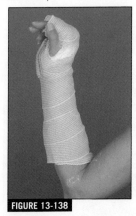

FIGURE 13-138

Technique 2: Two-Plaster, Dorsal-Ulnar Placement Modification

Equipment

1. Cast padding: 2 inches
2. Plaster: 2 inches
3. Elastic or self-adherent bandage: 3 inches

Basic Technique

1. The extremity is positioned and padded with cast padding as in technique 1.
2. Two overlapping plaster slabs are used instead of one.

Detailed Technique

1. Measure the length of the splint.
   a. Use the contralateral side.
   b. Take two measurements.
      (1) Measure one slab along the dorsum of the hand/forearm.
      (2) Measure another slab perpendicular to the first, starting at the dorsum of the hand and down the radial side of the hand/forearm.
2. Roll out the plaster.
   a. Two plaster slabs should be created, based on the aforementioned measurement.
   b. Each plaster slab should be 10 sheets thick.
3. Wrap the extremity in cast padding (see technique 1).
4. Prepare the plaster. Employ the usual technique of wetting and laminating (see Chapter 12).

5. Apply the plaster.
   a. Start by applying one slab along the dorsum of the fingers and forearm (Figure 13-139).
   b. Place a second slab along the dorsal side of the fingers and extending proximally down the volar-radial border of the forearm (Figure 13-140).
   c. The proximal part of the radial strip can be moved in a volar direction to help maintain the position of the splint.
6. Cover the plaster. Place cast padding over the top of the plaster to prevent the covering bandage from sticking to the plaster (Figure 13-141).
7. Mold the splint (see technique 1).
8. Perform a reduction maneuver if necessary.

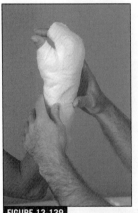

FIGURE 13-139

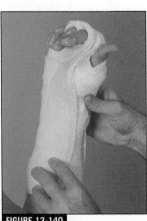

FIGURE 13-140

13

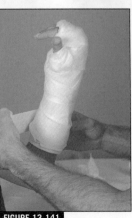

FIGURE 13-141

9. Definitively secure the splint with an elastic or self-adherent bandage (Figure 13-142).
   a. The bandage can be cut to minimize bulk between the long and ring fingers.
   b. The bandage can be cut to accommodate the thumb (Figure 13-143).
   c. Secure the end with silk tape if necessary.

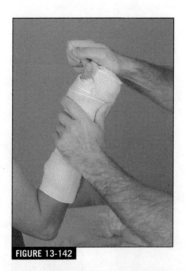

FIGURE 13-142

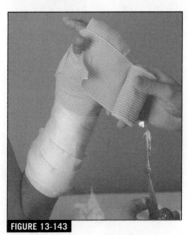

FIGURE 13-143

FINGER SPLINTS

Precautions

Beware of hyperextension at the IP joints in a dorsal splint; pressure necrosis is a common complication.

Pearls

1. Always place a finger splint on the dorsum of the finger unless a compelling reason exists not to.
2. For distal phalangeal injuries, a wraparound splint can help protect the distal phalanx from impact during daily activities (Figure 13-144).
3. For extensor tendon injuries at the PIP joint (central slip injury), splint only the PIP joint in extension, leaving the DIP free (Figure 13-145).
4. For extensor tendon injuries at the DIP joint (mallet injury), splint only the DIP joint in extension, leaving the PIP free (Figure 13-146).
   a. A wrap-around longitudinal strip of tape provides better control of the DIP joint (see Figure 13-144).
   b. A commercial stack splint also may be used for a mallet injury (Figure 13-147).

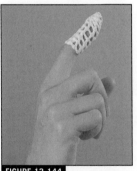

FIGURE 13-144

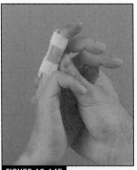

FIGURE 13-145

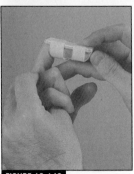

FIGURE 13-146

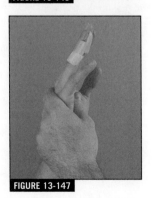

FIGURE 13-147

13

Equipment

1. Aluminum padded splint
2. ½-inch-wide silk tape

Basic Technique

1. Patient positioning:
   a. The patient is supine on a stretcher, standing, or sitting upright.
   b. The patient's elbow is supported on a table or stretcher and the hand is horizontal.
2. Landmarks:
   a. Digital condyles
   b. Metacarpal head
3. Where to start:
   a. PIP injury: just distal to the MP joint
   b. DIP injury: just distal to the PIP joint
   c. Thumb IP injury: just distal to the MP joint
   d. Middle phalanx fracture: just distal to the MP joint
   e. Distal phalanx fracture: just distal to the PIP joint
4. Where to finish:
   a. PIP injury: just proximal to the DIP joint
   b. DIP injury: at or just beyond the fingertip
   c. Thumb IP injury: at or just beyond the thumb tip
   d. Middle phalanx fracture: at or just beyond the fingertip
   e. Distal phalanx fracture: wrap around the fingertip ending on the volar surface just distal to the PIP joint
5. Where to mold:
   a. For dorsal dislocations or dorsally displaced/angulated fractures, incorporate a flexion bend to the aluminum foam splint.
   b. For volar dislocations or volarly displaced/angulated fractures, incorporate a very slight hyperextension bend to the aluminum foam splint.
   c. For dorsal tendon injuries, splint in slight hyperextension.
6. Steps:
   a. Position the patient.
   b. Perform a nerve block if indicated.
   c. Precut strips of tape to 3 inches in length.
   d. Prepare the aluminum foam splint.
   e. Perform a reduction maneuver.
   f. Apply the aluminum splint.
   g. Secure the splint in place with tape.
   h. Obtain postreduction views.

Detailed Technique

1. Position the patient so you have direct access to the fingers.
2. Perform a nerve block, if desired (see Chapter 1).
   a. An ulnar nerve block is reliable for the small finger.
   b. Use median and radial nerve blocks at the wrist for thumb dislocations.
   c. Digital blocks are sufficient for finger dislocations.
   d. Wait 10 to 15 minutes for the block to work.
3. Precut strips of ½-inch silk tape into 3-inch lengths.
4. Measure and cut the aluminum foam splint to size (Figure 13-148). Only splint the involved joint.
5. Trim away excess foam (Figure 13-149).

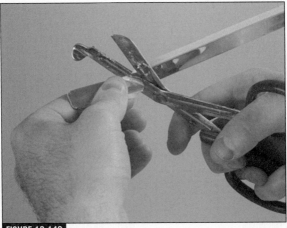

FIGURE 13-148

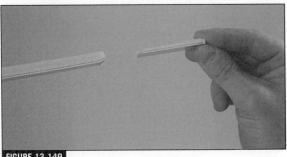

FIGURE 13-149

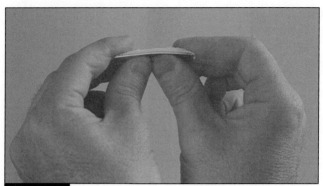

FIGURE 13-150

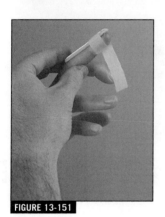

FIGURE 13-151

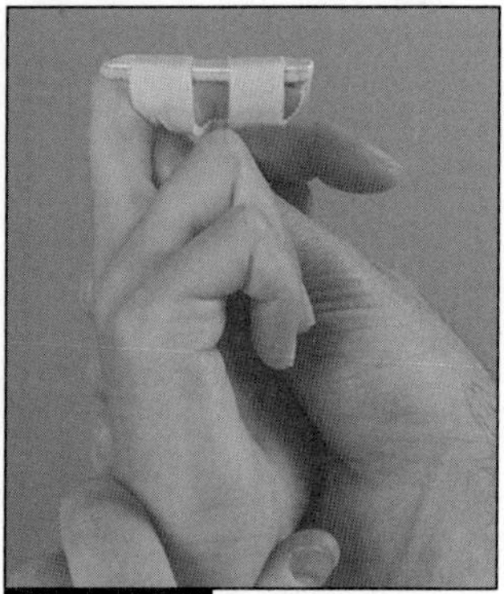

FIGURE 13-152

6. Contour the splint with appropriate bend (**Figure 13-150**).
   a. Dorsal dislocations (distal bone dislocates dorsally) should be splinted in flexion.
   b. Volar dislocations (distal bone dislocates volarly) should be splinted in extension.
7. Perform a reduction maneuver if indicated.
8. Place the padded aluminum splint.
   a. Hold the splint in place while applying tape circumferentially (**Figure 13-151**).
   b. Securing the distal end of the splint first is easiest (**Figure 13-152**).
9. Obtain postreduction films.

FINGER TAPE/STRAPS

Indications for Use

Finger MP, PIP, and DIP joint collateral ligament injuries

Precautions

Make sure that the tape or straps are not too tight to limit the vascularity of the digit.

Pearls

1. In general, two straps are better than one.
2. Place a piece of felt or gauze between two fingers if they are to be taped together for longer than a couple of days (Figure 13-153).
3. The relative thickness of the padding between the digits can be used to reduce angulated fractures (Figures 13-154 and 13-155).

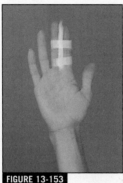

FIGURE 13-153

13

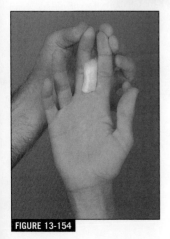

FIGURE 13-154

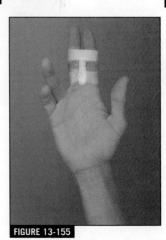

FIGURE 13-155

Equipment

1. Felt or gauze
2. ½-inch silk tape
3. Commercial buddy straps (optional)

Basic Technique

1. Patient positioning:
   a. The patient is supine on a stretcher, standing, or sitting upright.
   b. The patient's elbow is supported on a table or stretcher and the hand is horizontal.
2. Landmarks: digital condyles, metacarpal head
3. Where to start: between MP and PIP joints
4. Where to finish: between PIP and DIP joints
5. Where to mold: place a thicker amount of felt between the fingers proximally than distally to achieve a convergent reduction.
6. Steps:
   a. Position the patient.
   b. Perform a nerve block if indicated.
   c. Precut strips of tape 3 inches in length.
   d. Perform a reduction maneuver if indicated.
   e. Apply tape strips or buddy straps.
   f. Obtain postreduction views.

Detailed Technique

1. Position the patient so you have direct access to the fingers.
2. Perform a nerve block.
   a. An ulnar nerve block is reliable for the small finger.
   b. Digital blocks are sufficient for finger dislocations.
   c. Wait 10 to 15 minutes for the nerve block to work.
3. Precut strips of ½-inch silk tape into 3-inch lengths if using tape.
4. Perform a reduction maneuver if indicated.
5. Place felt padding or gauze between the fingers.

6. Apply buddy straps (Figures 13-156, 13-157, and 13-158) or tape.
7. Obtain postreduction films if indicated.

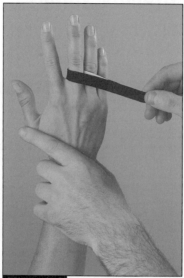

FIGURE 13-156

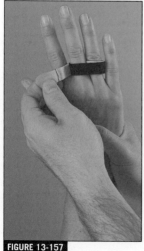

FIGURE 13-157

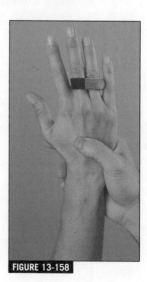

FIGURE 13-158

13

Chapter 14

Lower Extremity Splints and Casts

HIP SPICA CAST

Overview

1. The hip spica cast is one of the most difficult casts to apply.
2. The hip spica cast generally is composed of an abdominal portion attached to long leg casts, which is a so-called "double spica cast." When the unaffected extremity is placed into a thigh-only cast, the cast is termed a "1½ spica cast." A "single leg" hip spica cast is composed of an abdominal portion attached to a single long leg cast of the affected leg. All three types of spica casts have been shown to be successful in treating diaphyseal femoral fractures in children younger than 6 years.
3. The following points regarding the application of a hip spica cast are controversial:
   a. The type of spica cast that should be used (double, 1½, or single leg)
   b. Whether the foot should be included in the cast
   c. When to apply traction while casting
   d. Whether to apply the abdominal or the leg portion of the cast first
   e. Positioning of the extremity

Indications for Use

1. Pediatric femur fractures
2. General indications for type of spica cast:
   a. Double spica cast: concomitant pelvic or hip injury
   b. 1½ spica cast:
      (1) Proximal or mid diaphyseal femoral fractures
      (2) Older children
   c. Single leg spica cast: distal femoral fractures

Precautions

1. The following complications of hip spica casting may occur:
   a. Compartment syndrome has been reported in the 1½ spica cast with the hip and knee flexed to 90 degrees.
   b. Femoral and peroneal nerve palsy can occur, respectively, from excessive hip flexion and valgus molding over the fibular head.
   c. Skin breakdown and decubitus ulcers can occur.
   d. Superior mesenteric artery syndrome can occur from excessive thoracolumbar lordosis in the abdominal portion of the cast.

2. Close monitoring of the patient for complications is necessary during the first 2 weeks after application of the cast.
3. Some authors argue that initial femoral shortening greater than 2 cm is a contraindication for treatment with a spica cast.
4. Families caring for children with spica casts must contend with numerous psychosocial issues, such as transportation and bathing.

Pearls

1. We prefer a relaxed leg position with the knee at 60 degrees of flexion and the hip in 45 degrees of flexion rather than the traditional 90-90 position. An assistant should help the patient maintain this position throughout the application of the cast to avoid any bunching or creasing of the casting material.
2. Application of the cast can be performed in the emergency department with use of conscious sedation or in the operating room (OR) with use of general anesthesia.
3. Although they may not always be available, use of waterproof Gore-Tex pantaloons and a cast liner significantly improves the ability of the family to care for a child with a spica cast.
4. A broomstick, a twisted bar of fiberglass casting material, or some other connecting bar can be used to confer additional stability and strength to the spica cast.
5. Placing the spica table into a 10 degrees of reverse Trendelenburg position, either by tilting the operating table or by placing a block of wood under the spica table, allows the child's perineum to fit snugly against the perineal post of the spica table.

Equipment

1. Hip spica table
2. Two to four blue OR towels (or a towel folded so it is 2 inches thick)
3. A stockinette, with the size depending on the size of the child; typically, a 2-inch stockinette is used for the leg portions and either a 3-, 4-, or 6-inch stockinette is used for the abdominal portion.

14

4. A sawed-off portion of a broomstick or a fiberglass bar (Figures 14-1 and 14-2)
5. 4-inch cast padding
6. 4-inch fiberglass or plaster cast rolls

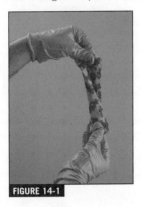

FIGURE 14-1

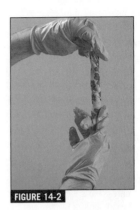

FIGURE 14-2

Basic Technique: 1½ Spica Cast

1. Patient positioning:
   a. The patient should be placed on the hip spica table (Figure 14-3).
      (1) The buttocks and perineum should be placed on the adjustable post.
      (2) The thoracic spine should sit on the table extension.
      (3) The shoulders and thorax should be on the platform portion of the table.
   b. The knee should be held at 60 degrees of flexion and the hip in 45 degrees of flexion. The hip should be abducted 20 to 30 degrees and the extremity should be externally rotated 15 degrees.

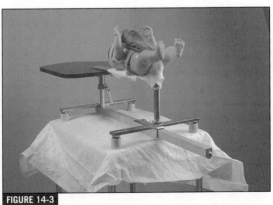

FIGURE 14-3

2. Where to start:
   a. A long leg cast is applied to the affected extremity starting with the foot.
   b. The foot should be included and placed in a neutral position.
3. Where to finish:
   a. The spica cast should extend proximally to the level of the rib cage.
4. Where to mold:
   a. A valgus mold should be placed at the fracture site.
5. Steps:
   a. Prepare a stockinette.
   b. Place the patient on the spica table.
   c. Position the stockinette.
   d. Place two to four blue OR towels on the abdomen under the stockinette to allow for abdominal excursion after application of the cast.
   e. Finish the cast edges.
   f. Apply the long leg cast on the affected extremity.
   g. Apply the abdominal portion of the spica cast and the contralateral thigh portion of the cast on the unaffected leg.
   h. Apply longitudinal traction to the affected extremity to achieve reduction.
   i. Incorporate the long leg cast into the abdominal cast.
   j. Mold the cast.
   k. Create a side strut for the affected extremity.
   l. Complete the cast.

Detailed Technique

1. Prepare a stockinette:
   a. Cut two pieces from a 2-inch stockinette:
      (1) One piece is for the long-leg portion of the spica cast, measuring from the inguinal crease to 2 inches beyond the foot.
      (2) One piece is for the contralateral thigh.
   b. Cut one piece from the 4-inch stockinette. This piece will be used for the abdominal portion of the spica cast and should measure from the nipples to the mid thigh.
2. Place the patient on the spica table. Have an assistant consistently hold the patient in the desired position.

14

3. Position the stockinette (Figure 14-4):
    a. Place the abdominal stockinette on the patient with the stockinette extending from the nipples to the mid thigh. Posteriorly, the stockinette should be placed over the spica table extension (i.e., the table should be in contact with the skin of the thoracic spine).
    b. Place the long-leg stockinette over the affected extremity and the unaffected-leg stockinette over the thigh of the contralateral leg.
4. Place two to four blue OR towels on the abdomen under the stockinette to allow for abdominal excursion after application of the cast.
5. Begin preparing the long leg cast on the affected extremity.

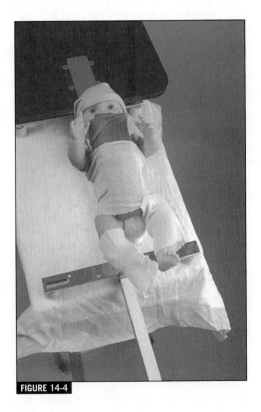

FIGURE 14-4

6. Wrap the extremity in cast padding (Figure 14-5).
   a. Start at the gluteal fold and circumferentially wrap distally to the area immediately above the lateral malleolus.
      (1) Use a standard 50% overlap technique (see Chapter 12).
      (2) Two layers of wrapping are sufficient.
   b. Span the joint line with cast padding at the anterior aspect of the tibiotalar joint (see aforementioned precautions for the long leg cast).
   c. Return to the lateral malleolus and wrap over this area.
   d. Continue distally to around the foot. Do not cover the heel at this point.
   e. Once sufficient padding has been wrapped around the malleoli and the foot, the heel can be addressed.
   f. Tear strips of cast padding and lay them on top of the heel (Figure 14-6). Repeat several times to ensure sufficient padding.

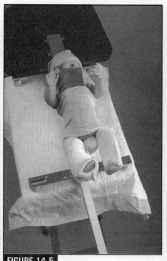

FIGURE 14-5

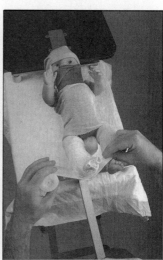

FIGURE 14-6

7. Create a cast padding cuff (see Chapter 12) for the metatarsal heads. This cuff should form a "V" at the lateral aspect of the foot to allow for the cascade of the digits (Figure 14-7).
8. Wrap the abdomen in cast padding (Figure 14-8). Ensure that the anterior superior iliac spine, posterior superior iliac spine, and sacrum are very well padded.
9. Wrap the contralateral thigh in cast padding. Start immediately proximal to the popliteal fossa and continue proximally to the gluteal fold.

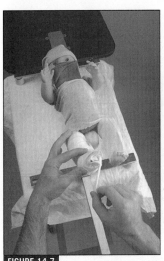

FIGURE 14-7

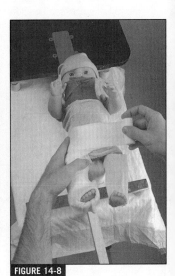

FIGURE 14-8

10. Create a cuff of cast padding (Figure 14-9) and place it over the most distal part of the rib cage.
11. Create a cuff of cast padding.
    a. Place the cuff over the distal portion of the thigh.
    b. The knee should be able to bend to 90 degrees without impediment from the cast.
12. Finish the cast edges (Figure 14-10). All exposed areas should have the stockinette pulled up and folded over the cast padding.
13. Pay particular attention to the perineal portion of the cast.

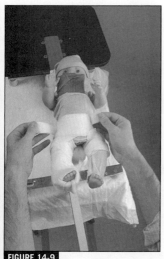
FIGURE 14-9

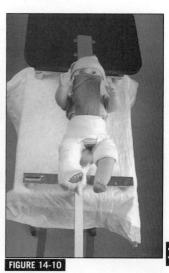
FIGURE 14-10

14

14. Apply cast material as for a long leg cast.
    a. Start distally at the metatarsal heads and extend proximally to the mid thigh.
    b. Ensure that a significant amount of stockinette and cast padding remains to the level of the gluteal fold (Figure 14-11).
    c. Be vigilant about the position of the foot.
15. Begin application of the abdominal portion of the spica cast and the contralateral thigh portion of the cast for the unaffected leg.
    a. Begin proximally at the level of the abdominal cuff of cast padding and continue distally.
    b. Carefully incorporate only the unaffected leg into the abdominal portion, using a figure-of-8 technique around the hip (Figure 14-12).
    c. Do not yet incorporate the long leg cast of the affected extremity.
16. Apply longitudinal traction to the affected extremity to achieve reduction if necessary.

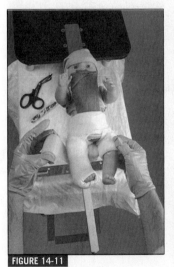

FIGURE 14-11

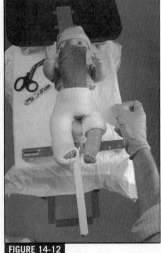

FIGURE 14-12

17. Incorporate the long leg cast into the abdominal cast (**Figure 14-13**).
    a. Use a figure-of-8 technique.
    b. Ensure that the perineum remains exposed.
18. Mold the cast (**Figure 14-14**):
    a. Place one palm on the lateral aspect of the thigh immediately proximal to the fracture site.
    b. Place the other palm on the medial aspect distal to the fracture site.
    c. Mold the cast into valgus.
19. Create a side strut for the affected extremity if plaster is being used.
    a. Take a roll of plaster and create a splint that is 10 layers thick extending from the mid abdomen to the mid thigh.
    b. Apply the splint obliquely along the inferior lateral buttock area to act as a strut.

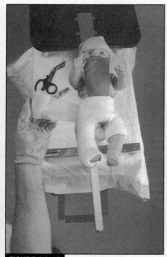

FIGURE 14-13

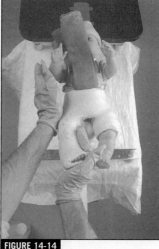

FIGURE 14-14

14

20. Apply a broomstick or bar of fiberglass to span both legs. Incorporate the strut and the bar into the spica cast with an additional roll of fiberglass (Figure 14-15).
21. Complete the cast (Figure 14-16):
    a. Use colored fiberglass for a "Hollywood roll" if desired.
    b. Remove towels from the abdomen.
    c. Remove the child from the spica table.
    d. Trim away any excess casting material.

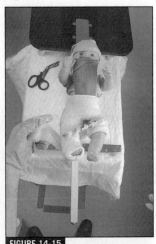

FIGURE 14-15

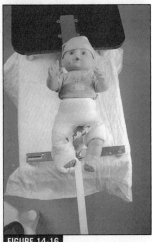

FIGURE 14-16

LONG-LEG SPLINT

Overview

The design of the long-leg splint is identical to that of the AO splint described later, with a posterior slab and a stirrup, except that each of the slabs traverses the knee and extends to the upper thigh.

Indications for Use

1. Tibial shaft fracture
2. Tibial plateau fracture
3. Distal femur fracture

Precautions

1. As in any other splint that immobilizes the ankle and foot, the position of the foot within the splint is of paramount importance. Do not allow the foot to be in equinus except in the case of very distal tibial shaft fractures where dorsiflexion results in extension at the fracture site.
2. The long-leg splint is placed with the knee in 20 to 30 degrees of flexion.
3. Given the propensity for tibial shaft fractures to become very swollen and the associated high risk for compartment syndrome, Jones' cotton typically is used.

Pearls

1. Before starting, ensure that adequate analgesia has been achieved, either with intravenous opioids or conscious sedation.
2. The long-leg splint is one of the most difficult splints to apply; having the aid of two assistants facilitates the process. If help is not available, use either the technique described below or this alternative method to elevate the limb (Figure 14-17):
   a. Have the patient lay supine on a stretcher with side rails.
   b. Raise both side rails.
   c. Take two rolls of 6-inch rolled gauze and unravel them completely.
   d. Lay one roll of rolled gauze under the patient's thigh and the other under the calf, with equal lengths on each side of the limb.

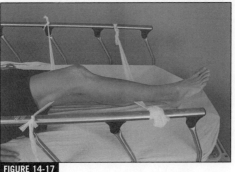

FIGURE 14-17

e. Start with the roll under the calf:
  (1) Tie one end to the side rail.
  (2) Pull on the other side until the gauze is taut and the limb is
      elevated; tie the end to the side rail.
  f. Repeat with the roll under the thigh.
3. It is recommended that cool water be used (to delay plaster setting) and
   that all three plaster slabs be prepared in water prior to application of
   the splint. This approach reduces the amount of time the patient needs
   to be elevated and thus reduces patient discomfort. It also reduces the
   amount of work that needs to be done by the assistants.
4. For high-energy injuries, we prefer to use Jones' cotton in place of
   regular cotton cast padding.
5. Use of a "mega-ACE" bandage that is 11 yards long makes securing
   this splint much more manageable because it eliminates the need for
   multiple elastic bandages.
6. Premade 45-inch plaster slabs typically are an appropriate length for all
   three slabs necessary for this splint.

Equipment

1. 4- or 6-inch stockinette
2. Jones' cotton and/or 6-inch cast padding
3. 4-, 5-, or 6-inch plaster
4. 6-inch elastic or self-adherent bandage
5. 2-inch silk tape

Basic Technique

1. Patient positioning:
   a. Supine on a stretcher
2. Where to start:
   a. Upper thigh both medially and laterally
3. Where to finish:
   a. Distal aspect of foot; may include the toes
4. Where to mold:
   a. Supracondylar region and/or supramalleolar region to prevent
      migration of the splint distalward
5. Steps:
   a. Measure the length of the splint.
   b. Roll out the plaster.
   c. Prepare the plaster in the usual fashion.
   d. Position the patient.
   e. Apply Jones' cotton or other cast padding.
   f. Apply slabs of plaster.
   g. Apply a second layer of cast padding.
   h. Overwrap with an elastic bandage.
   i. Mold the splint.

Detailed Technique

1. Measure the length of the splint using plaster (Figures 14-18 and 14-19):
   a. Use the contralateral uninjured side if necessary.
   b. A single measurement will be taken using the lateral aspect.
   c. Measure from the medial malleolus, circle around the foot, and extend until the upper aspect of the lateral thigh is reached.
2. Roll out the plaster.
   a. The plaster slab should be 10 to 12 sheets thick.
   b. Alternatively, use 45 × 5 inch prefabricated slabs.
3. Prepare the plaster in the usual fashion. Use the standard technique of wetting and laminating (see Chapter 12).
   a. Use water that is slightly cooler than that used for other splints.
   b. Hang the plaster strips from the stretcher or lay them out on a bed sheet.

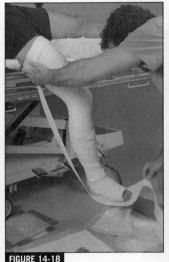

FIGURE 14-18

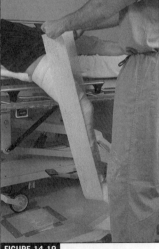

FIGURE 14-19

4. Place a padded crutch beneath the mattress on the stretcher so that only a foot of the top of the stretcher remains visible (Figure 14-20).
5. Position the patient:
   a. The patient is supine with his or her pelvis halfway onto the crutch (Figure 14-21). Make sure the patient and the crutch are secure.

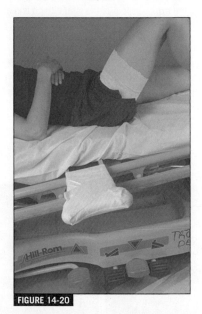

FIGURE 14-20

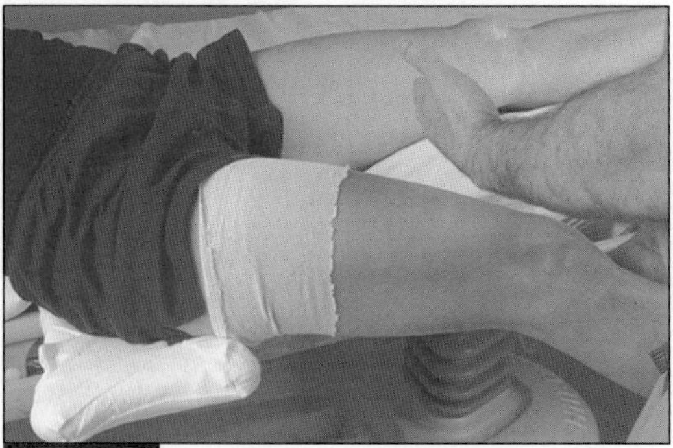

FIGURE 14-21

b. Allow the limb to hang down, or support it by placing the patient's foot on your thigh (Figure 14-22). If assistants are available, they can elevate the limb.

6. Apply Jones' cotton or regular cast padding (Figure 14-23):
   a. If using Jones' cotton, start at metatarsal heads and wrap in a circumferential fashion proximally to the mid thigh with minimal overlap.
   b. If using standard padding, begin proximally or distally depending on your preference.

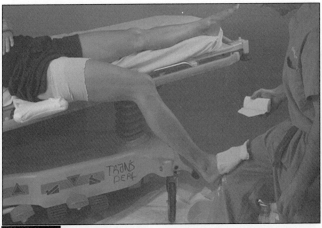

FIGURE 14-22

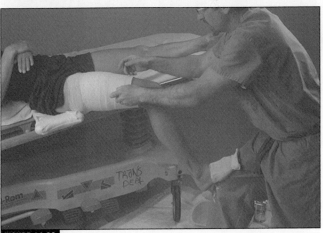

FIGURE 14-23

7. Apply the splint.
   a. Begin with the posterior slab:
      (1) Start at the foot and extend proximally.
      (2) Provisionally secure the splint with cast padding at the knee and then the thigh (Figure 14-24).
      (3) Fold down any excess splint.
   b. Apply the lateral and medial wraparound slab:
      (1) Start proximally at the upper thigh and extend distally (Figure 14-25).

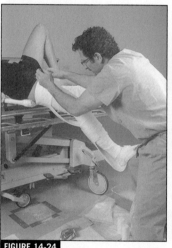

FIGURE 14-24

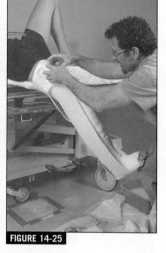

FIGURE 14-25

    (2) Provisionally secure the splint with cast padding at the thigh and
        then at the knee.
    (3) Overwrap with cast padding (Figure 14-26).
8. Perform a reduction maneuver if required.
9. Definitively secure the splint with an ACE wrap (Figures 14-27
   and 14-28):
   a. Start at the foot and extend proximally.
   b. Secure the end with silk tape.

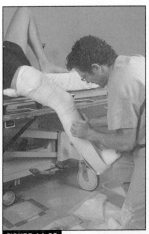

FIGURE 14-26

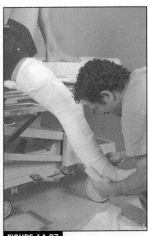

FIGURE 14-27

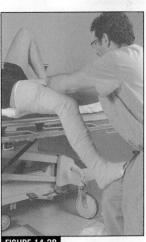

FIGURE 14-28

10. Mold the splint:
    a. At this point, assistants are no longer necessary.
    b. The limb is taken by the surgeon, the foot is placed on the thigh, and an axial load is applied to ensure the foot is not in equinus.
       (1) This position naturally places the knee at approximately 30 degrees of flexion.
       (2) Perform either a supramalleolar mold (Figure 14-29) or a supracondylar mold (Figure 14-30) or both.

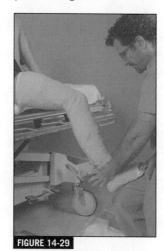

FIGURE 14-29

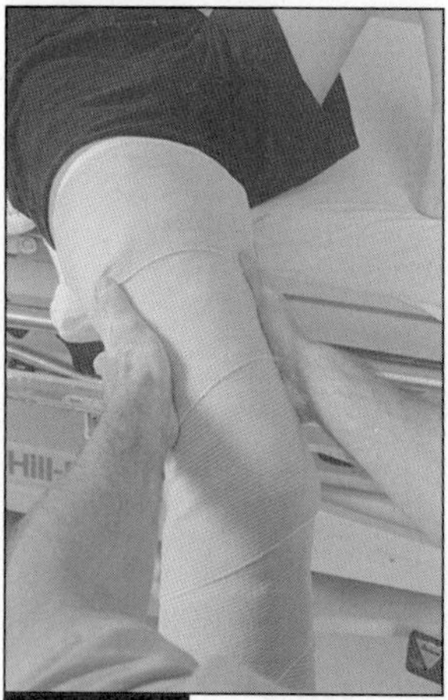

FIGURE 14-30

LONG LEG CAST

Indications for Use

Tibial shaft fractures

Precautions

1. The position of the foot in the plaster is of paramount importance.
   a. The equinus position is defined as a foot plantarflexed beyond neutral.
   b. If the foot is left in an equinus position for a prolonged period, the Achilles tendon becomes contracted and ankle stiffness ensues.
2. At the anterior aspect of the ankle, do not allow edges of the cast padding to lay immediately within the joint line.
   a. Allowing edges of the cast padding to lay immediately within the joint line will create wrinkling and can lead to skin breakdown in this very fragile area.
   b. Span the area by having the mid-point of the cast padding roll directly over the ankle flexion crease; by doing so, the cast padding will be slightly tented above the joint line and will not be in direct contact with the skin, thus reducing the risk of skin breakdown.

Pearls

1. Before starting, ensure that adequate analgesia has been achieved, either with intravenous opioids or conscious sedation. Occasionally, long leg casts are placed under general anesthesia in the operating room to allow for fluoroscopic-guided reduction and maximum patient comfort.
2. Two techniques may be used for application of a long leg cast:
   a. Application of a short leg cast and then completion of the upper leg portion is the easiest technique to perform.
   b. Application of a long leg cast by starting at the thigh and continuing distally in one sitting creates the strongest cast.
3. Application of a long leg cast is difficult; having the aid of an assistant makes it easier. If an assistant is unavailable, use the following technique:
   a. Carefully pad a standard walking crutch.
   b. Lower the guard rail on the stretcher.
   c. Place the crutch under the mattress of the stretcher at the level of the hip, with one third sticking out on the affected side (see Figure 14-20).
   d. Have the patient rest his or her buttocks on the crutch.
   e. Position the limb with your leg.

14

Equipment

1. 4- or 6-inch stockinette
2. 4- or 6 inch cast padding.
3. 4 or 6-inch plaster or fiberglass

Basic Technique

1. Patient positioning:
   a. The patient is sitting off the end of the bed.
   b. Ensure that at least half of the thigh is off the bed to allow for space between the leg and the bed.
   c. The knee is flexed 10 to 30 degrees and the ankle is in a neutral position.
2. Where to start:
   a. Metatarsal heads
3. Where to finish:
   a. Upper thigh
4. Where to mold:
   a. Supracondylar femur
   b. Supramalleolar tibia
5. Steps:
   a. Prepare a stockinette.
   b. Position the stockinette.
   c. Position the patient.
   d. Wrap the extremity in cast padding.
   e. Create and apply cuffs of cast padding (see Chapter 12).
   f. Fold down the end of the stockinette at the foot and thigh.
   g. Prepare plaster.
   h. Apply plaster.
   i. Allow the cast to dry before lowering the leg.

Detailed Technique

1. Prepare a stockinette by cutting two pieces:
   a. One piece is for the proximal portion at the thigh.
   b. One piece is for the distal portion at the foot.
2. Position the stockinette (see Figure 14-22):
   a. Place one stockinette over the proximal thigh.
   b. Place the other stockinette with equal lengths centered over the metatarsal heads.

3. Position the patient.
    a. Place a padded crutch beneath the mattress on the stretcher so that only 1 foot of the top of the stretcher remains visible (see Figure 14-20).
    b. The patient is supine with his or her pelvis halfway onto the crutch (see Figure 14-21). Make sure the patient and the crutch are secure to prevent a fall.
    c. Allow the limb to hang down or support it by placing the patient's foot on your thigh (see Figure 14-22). If available, an assistant can elevate the limb.
    d. If the patient is anesthetized, bring the patient to the edge of the bed and drape the extremity over the side with an assistant holding the leg.
4. Wrap the extremity in cast padding.
    a. Start at the thigh and circumferentially wrap distally (see Figure 14-23).
        (1) Use a standard 50% overlap technique (see Chapter 12).
        (2) Two layers of wrapping are sufficient.
    b. Span the joint line with cast padding at the posterior aspect of the knee (see aforementioned precautions) (Figure 14-31).

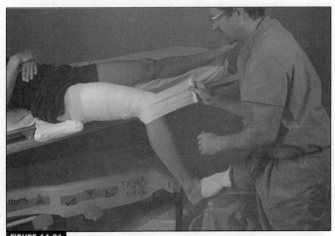

FIGURE 14-31

14

c. Continue distally to around the foot:
  (1) Span the joint line with cast padding at the ankle (see
      aforementioned precautions) (Figure 14-32).
  (2) Do not cover the heel at this point (Figure 14-33).
d. Once sufficient padding has been wrapped around the malleoli and
   the foot, the heel can be addressed.

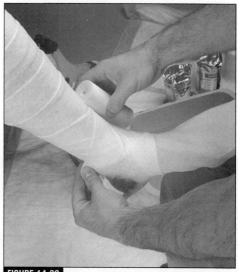

FIGURE 14-32

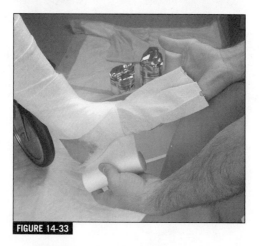

FIGURE 14-33

e. Tear 4-inch strips of cast padding and lay them on top of the heel (Figure 14-34). Repeat several times to ensure sufficient padding.

5. Create a cast padding cuff (see Chapter 12) for the metatarsal heads (Figure 14-35). This cuff should form a V at the lateral aspect of the foot to allow for the cascade of the digits.

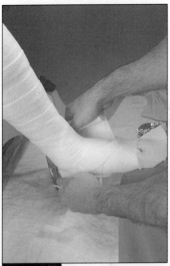

FIGURE 14-34

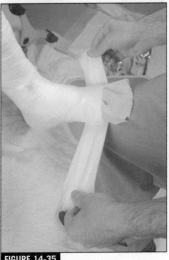

FIGURE 14-35

6. Fold down the end of the stockinette at the foot (Figure 14-36) and thigh (Figure 14-37).
7. Prepare the plaster. Use the standard technique of wetting and laminating (see Chapter 12).

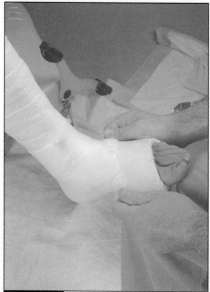

FIGURE 14-36

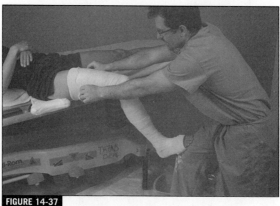

FIGURE 14-37

8. Apply the plaster.
   a. Start at the thigh and work distally (Figure 14-38). Use the standard technique of laminating while rolling (see Chapter 12).
   b. Be vigilant about the position of the foot.
   c. The foot can easily fall into equinus (Figure 14-39).
   d. Additional thickness over the plantar aspect of the foot can be achieved by adding several precut strips.
9. Allow the cast to dry before lowering the leg.

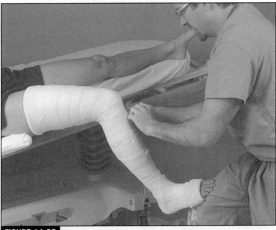

FIGURE 14-38

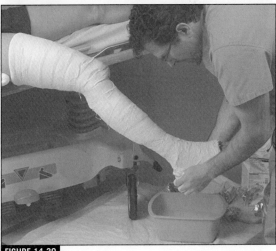

FIGURE 14-39

CYLINDER CAST

Indications for Use

1. Patellar fractures
2. Patellar dislocations

Precautions

Be sure to pad the malleoli thickly to avoid pressure sores on the ankle and to limit distal migration of the cast (Figure 14-40).

Pearls

Have the patient stand with his or her knee in slight flexion, sufficiently straight to walk on but bent enough to be comfortable.

Equipment

1. Stockinette
2. Cast padding
3. Plaster

Basic Technique

1. Patient positioning:
   a. The patient is standing.
   b. The knee is flexed 5 to 10 degrees and the ankle is plantigrade on the floor.
2. Where to start: over the malleoli
3. Where to finish: upper thigh
4. Where to mold: supracondylar femur

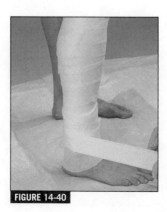

FIGURE 14-40

5. Steps:
   a. Prepare a stockinette.
   b. Position the stockinette.
   c. Position the patient.
   d. Wrap the extremity in cast padding.
   e. Create and apply cast padding cuffs (see Chapter 12).
   f. Fold down the end of the stockinette at the ankle and thigh.
   g. Prepare the plaster.
   h. Apply the plaster.
   i. Apply the mold.

Detailed Technique

1. Prepare a stockinette by cutting it into two pieces:
   a. One piece is for the proximal portion at the thigh.
   b. One piece is for the distal portion at the lower leg.
2. Position the patient and place the stockinette segments (Figure 14-41):
   a. Place one stockinette over the proximal thigh.
   b. Place the other over the malleoli.
3. Wrap the extremity in cast padding.
   a. Start at either end and wrap circumferentially (Figure 14-42).
      (1) Use a standard 50% overlap technique (see Chapter 12).
      (2) Two layers of wrapping are sufficient.

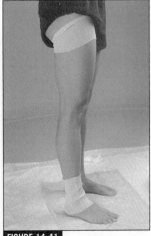

FIGURE 14-41

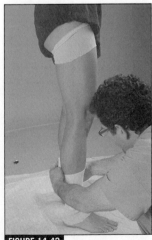

FIGURE 14-42

b. Span the joint line with cast padding at the posterior aspect of the knee (see aforementioned precautions) (Figure 14-43).
c. Apply a thick cuff of cast padding at the ankle (Figure 14-44).

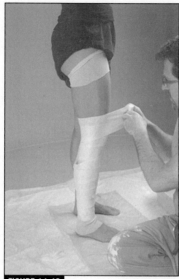

FIGURE 14-43

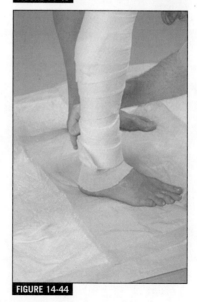

FIGURE 14-44

4. Create a cast padding cuff (see Chapter 12) for the malleoli (Figure 14-45).
5. Fold down the end of the stockinette at the ankle (Figure 14-46) and thigh (Figure 14-47).
6. Prepare the plaster. Use the standard technique of wetting and laminating (see Chapter 12).

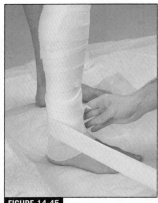

FIGURE 14-45

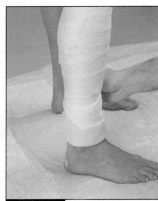

FIGURE 14-46

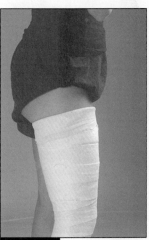

FIGURE 14-47

14

7. Apply the plaster:
   a. Start at the thigh and work distally (Figure 14-48).
   b. Use the standard technique of laminating while rolling (see Chapter 12).
   c. Be vigilant about the position of the knee.
   d. Additional thickness behind the knee can be achieved by adding several precut strips.
8. Apply the mold (Figure 14-49).

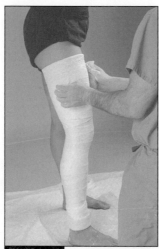

FIGURE 14-48

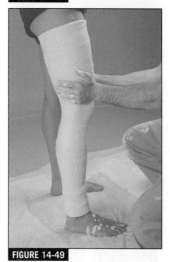

FIGURE 14-49

AO SPLINT

Overview

1. The AO splint is constructed with three plaster slabs:
   a. A medial slab and a lateral slab in a J-type configuration
   b. A posterior slab in an L-type configuration
2. The AO splint also can be constructed with two plaster slabs:
   a. A U-type slab substitutes for the two J-type slabs.
   b. The posterior slab in an L-type configuration remains unchanged.
3. The technique described for this splint is application without the Quigley maneuver. If the Quigley maneuver is used, the splint is applied in the same fashion but the patient is supine on a stretcher.

Indications for Use

1. Ankle fractures
2. Pilon fractures

Precautions

1. The position of the foot in the plaster is of paramount importance.
   a. The equinus position is defined as a foot plantarflexed beyond neutral.
   b. If the foot is left in an equinus position for a prolonged period, the Achilles tendon becomes contracted and ankle stiffness ensues.
2. Swelling is a significant concern for ankle fractures; the degree of swelling often worsens after 2 to 3 days.
   a. A bulky cotton padding (variously known as Sir Robert Jones' cotton, Bulky Jones cotton, and Red Cross cotton) can be applied below the plaster slabs to allow the splint to accommodate the swelling.
   b. The medial and lateral slabs should be kept slightly posterior on the leg to prevent them from joining at the anterior aspect. If they join both posteriorly and anteriorly, this position creates a circumferential cast construct.

14

Pearls

1. Many ankle fractures are reduced with use of the Quigley maneuver. By having the patient keep his or her leg in extension during the Quigley maneuver, the ankle will naturally be kept out of equinus.
2. For instances in which a reduction maneuver is not used, two techniques can be used to keep the foot out of equinus:
   a. The patient may lie prone with his or her knee bent to 90 degrees. Gravity will aid but not completely prevent equinus.
      (1) To completely prevent equinus with the patient prone, use the following technique:
         (a) Cut a 6-foot-long piece of 4- or 6-inch stockinette.
         (b) Put the stockinette on the patient up to the mid thigh.
         (c) Have the patient lie prone and flex his or her knee to 90 degrees.
         (d) Tie the loose end to the end of the bed so the ankle is out of equinus.
         (e) Apply the splint.
         (f) Once the splint is completely applied, cut the stockinette close to the ends of the splint and tuck the ends under the ACE wrap.
      (2) This technique typically is used for a child.
   b. The patient is kept supine while the splint is applied. The hip is slightly flexed, the knee is bent to 90 degrees, and the foot is placed on the surgeon's chest. Axial pressure is applied until the plaster has set. This technique typically is used with unconscious patients.
3. When applying Jones' cotton, splitting it in half width-wise is useful. Halving the thickness of the cotton by splitting it longitudinally also is possible.
4. Using cool water and preparing all three plaster slabs in water prior to application of the splint is the easiest technique to use and eliminates the need for an assistant.
5. When applying the medial and lateral slabs, always start at the proximal aspect of the limb. If the splint is long, it can simply be carried up the other side.

Equipment

1. 4-inch stockinette
2. 4- or 6-inch cast padding
3. 4- or 6-inch plaster
4. 4- or 6-inch elastic or self-adherent bandage
5. 2-inch silk tape

Basic Technique

1. Patient positioning:
   a. If the Quigley maneuver is used: The patient is supine on a stretcher with his or her leg elevated by traction.
   b. If the supine or sitting technique is used: The patient is supine or sitting on a stretcher with the knee and lower leg off the bed.
   c. If the prone technique is used: The patient is prone on a stretcher with the knee flexed to 90 degrees.
2. Where to start:
   a. Metatarsal heads
3. Where to finish:
   a. Tibial tubercle
4. Where to mold for ankle fracture:
   a. Distal to the lateral malleolus over the calcaneus
   b. Immediately proximal to the medial malleolus
5. Steps:
   a. Measure the length of the splint using plaster.
   b. Roll out the plaster.
   c. Roll out the cast padding.
   d. Position the patient.
   e. Perform a modified Quigley maneuver to reduce the fracture if necessary.
   f. Apply Jones' cotton, if desired.
   g. Prepare the plaster in the usual fashion.
   h. Apply plaster slabs.
   i. Overwrap the plaster slabs with cast padding.
   j. Definitively secure the splint with an elastic or self-adherent bandage.
   k. Perform molding and reduction if necessary.

14

Detailed Technique: Application Sitting

1. Perform an intra-articular ankle block, if desired (see Chapter 6).
2. Measure the length of the splint (Figures 14-50 and 14-51):
   a. Use the contralateral side if necessary.
   b. Two different measurements will be taken: a wrap-around U splint measurement and a posterior measurement.
      (1) Note that two different plaster slabs will be used: one U slab and one posterior slab.
      (2) Posterior:
         (a) Start immediately distal to the popliteal fossa.
         (b) End at the metatarsal heads.
      (3) Lateral:
         (a) Start immediately proximal to the fibular head.
         (b) End at the medial arch of the foot.

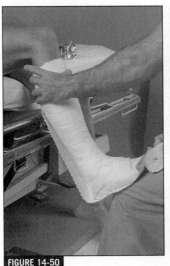
FIGURE 14-50

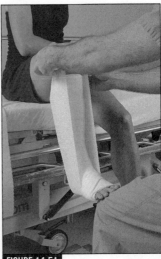
FIGURE 14-51

3. Roll out the plaster.
   a. The plaster slab should be 10 to 12 sheets thick.
   b. Two different slabs will be created, with the U slab being approximately 25% longer than the posterior slab.
4. Position the patient:
   a. The patient should be supine or sitting with the knee and lower leg off the bed and the ball of the foot resting on your knee or thigh.
   b. Create toe traps using rolled gauze if using modified Quigley traction (see Chapter 11).
   c. Attach the gauze to the patient's toes using a dual-ring construct:
      (1) Make a loop of gauze.
      (2) Place the loop between the web space of the great toe and second toe.
      (3) While holding one side of the gauze taught, place your other hand into the loop.
      (4) Spread your fingers and pull upward.
      (5) Hook each side around the great toe and second finger.
      (6) Pull the free end taut.
5. Apply cast padding (or Jones' cotton, if desired) (Figures 14-52, 14-53, and 14-54):
   a. Start at either end and wrap in a circumferential fashion from the metatarsal heads to the level of the fibular head and tibial tubercle.
   b. Because of the thickness of the Jones' cotton, very little overlap is necessary.

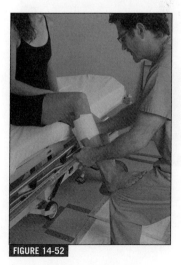

FIGURE 14-52

14

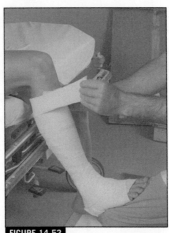

FIGURE 14-53

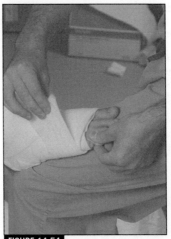

FIGURE 14-54

6. Prepare the plaster in the usual fashion.
   a. Use the standard technique of wetting and laminating (see Chapter 12).
   b. Prepare both slabs at the same time before application.
   c. Water that is slightly cooler than that used for other procedures should be used.
7. Apply the plaster slabs.
   a. Begin with the posterior slab (Figure 14-55).
      (1) Start at foot and extend proximally.
      (2) Fold down excess at the knee if it is encountered.
   b. Apply the U slab (Figure 14-56).
      (1) Start proximally at the fibular head and extend distally.

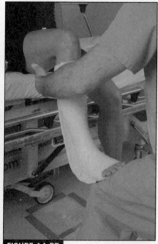

FIGURE 14-55

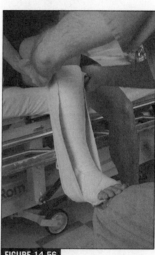

FIGURE 14-56

254 Splints and Casts

8. Overwrap with a single layer of cast padding (Figures 14-57 and 14-58).
9. Definitively secure the splint with an ACE wrap (Figure 14-59):
    a. Start at either end and advance to the other end.
    b. Secure the end with silk tape or Velcro.

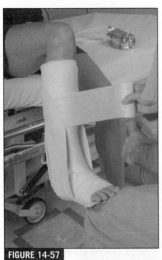
FIGURE 14-57

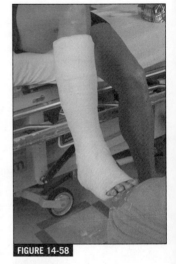
FIGURE 14-58

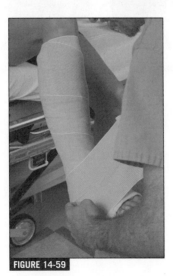
FIGURE 14-59

10. Perform molding:
    a. Ankle fracture (see Chapter 11)
    b. If no reduction is necessary, apply supramalleolar molding
       (Figure 14-60).

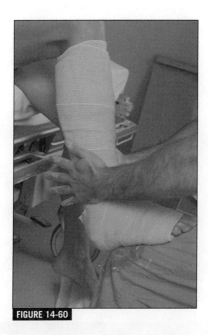

FIGURE 14-60

14

SHORT-LEG CAST

Indications for Use

1. Ankle fractures (nonacute)
2. Achilles tendon rupture (in equinus)

Precautions

1. The position of the foot in the plaster is of paramount importance.
   a. The equinus position is defined as a foot plantarflexed beyond neutral.
   b. If the foot is left in an equinus position for a prolonged period, the Achilles tendon becomes contracted and ankle stiffness ensues.
   c. When a short leg cast is used for an Achilles tendon rupture, 10 to 15 degrees of equinus is desirable, and an optional heel can be built into the cast to facilitate weight bearing in the cast while maintaining equinus (Figures 14-61 and 14-62).

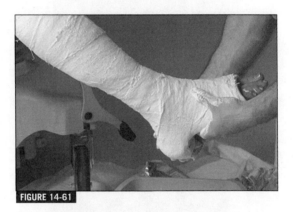
FIGURE 14-61

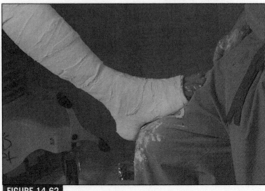
FIGURE 14-62

2. At the anterior aspect of the ankle, do not allow edges of cast padding to lay immediately within the joint line.
   a. Allowing edges of cast padding to lay immediately within the joint line will create wrinkling and can lead to skin breakdown in this very fragile area.
   b. Span the area by having the mid-point of the cast padding roll directly over the ankle flexion crease; by doing so, the cast padding will be slightly tented above the joint line and will not be in direct contact with the skin, thus reducing the risk of skin breakdown.

Pearls

1. Raise the stretcher as high as it will go to make application of the cast easier.
2. Keeping the foot out of equinus sometimes can be difficult. If no reduction is necessary, placing the patient in a prone position can facilitate proper positioning of the ankle:
   a. The patient may lay prone with his or her knee bent to 90 degrees. Gravity will aid but not completely prevent equinus.
   b. To prevent equinus with the patient prone, use the following technique:
      (1) Cut a 6-foot-long piece of a 4- or 6-inch stockinette.
      (2) Put the stockinette on the patient up to the mid thigh.
      (3) Have the patient lay prone and flex his or her knee to 90 degrees.
      (4) Tie the loose end to the end of the bed so the ankle is out of equinus.
      (5) Apply the splint.
      (6) Once the splint is completely applied, cut the stockinette close to the ends of the splint and tuck the ends under the elastic bandage.

Equipment

1. 4-inch stockinette
2. 4- or 6-inch cast padding
3. 4- to 6-inch plaster or fiberglass

Basic Technique

1. Patient positioning:
   a. The patient is sitting off the end of the bed. Ensure that at least half the thigh is off the bed to allow for space between the leg and the bed.
   b. Alternatively, the patient may be placed prone with the knee flexed to 90 degrees.
2. Where to start:
   a. Metatarsal heads
3. Where to finish:
   a. Tibial tubercle

14

4. Where to mold:
    a. No reduction: supramalleolar mold
    b. Ankle fracture:
        (1) Distal to the lateral malleolus over the calcaneus
        (2) Immediately proximal to the medial malleolus
5. Steps:
    a. Position the patient.
    b. Prepare a stockinette.
    c. Position the stockinette.
    d. Wrap the extremity in cast padding.
    e. Create two cuffs of cast padding (see Chapter 12).
    f. Fold down the two ends of the stockinette.
    g. Prepare the cast material.
    h. Apply the cast material.
    i. Apply molding or a reduction as needed.
    j. Split the cast if necessary.

Detailed Technique

1. Position the patient (Figure 14-63):
    a. The patient is sitting upright and the leg is freely off the end of the bed.
    b. Make sure the patient is sitting far enough forward so there is sufficient room between the posterior calf and the end of the bed.
2. Prepare a stockinette by cutting it into two pieces:
    a. One piece is for the proximal portion at the knee.
    b. One piece is for the distal portion at the foot.

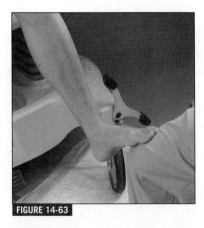

FIGURE 14-63

3. Position the stockinette segments (Figure 14-64):
   a. Place one stockinette segment over the knee with equal lengths on either side.
   b. Place the other segment with equal lengths centered over the metatarsal heads.
4. Wrap the extremity in cast padding:
   a. Start at the level of the tibial tubercle and circumferentially wrap distally to the area immediately above the lateral malleolus.
      (1) Use a standard 50% overlap technique (see Chapter 12).
      (2) Two layers of wrapping are sufficient.
   b. Span the joint line with cast padding at the anterior aspect of the ankle (see aforementioned precautions) (Figure 14-65).
   c. Return to the lateral malleolus and wrap over this area.
   d. Continue distally to around the foot (see Figure 14-33). Do not cover the heel at this point.

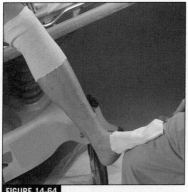

FIGURE 14-64

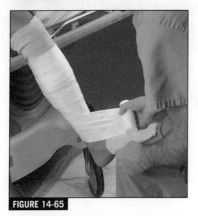

FIGURE 14-65

14

  e. Once sufficient padding has been wrapped around the malleoli and the foot, the heel can be addressed.

  f. Tear 4-inch strips of cast padding and lay them on top of the heel (Figure 14-66). Repeat several times to ensure sufficient padding.

5. Create two cast padding cuffs (see Chapter 12):

  a. Metatarsal heads (see Figure 14-35): This cuff should form a "V" at the lateral aspect of the foot to allow for the cascade of the digits.

  b. Tibial tubercle (Figure 14-67): This cuff can be circular.

6. Fold down the two ends of stockinette (see Figure 14-36).

7. Prepare the plaster. Use the standard technique of wetting and laminating (see Chapter 12).

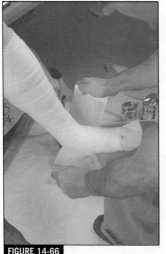

FIGURE 14-66

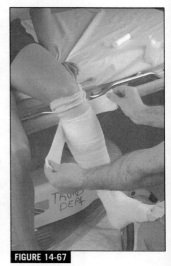

FIGURE 14-67

8. Apply the plaster.
   a. Start at the tibial tubercle and work distally (Figure 14-68). Use the standard technique of laminating while rolling (see Chapter 12).
      (1) Be vigilant about the position of the foot (Figure 14-69).
      (2) Additional thickness over the plantar aspect of the foot can be achieved by adding several precut strips, if desired.
9. Apply molding or perform a reduction as needed.
10. Split the cast if necessary.

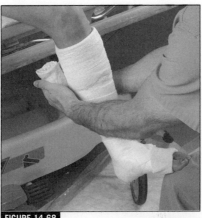

FIGURE 14-68

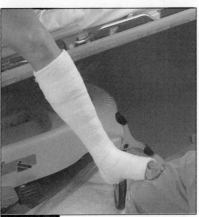

FIGURE 14-69

PATELLAR TENDON BEARING (PTB) CAST

Indications for Use
Low tibial shaft fractures

Precautions
1. The position of the foot in the plaster is of paramount importance.
   a. The equinus position is defined as a foot plantarflexed beyond neutral.
   b. If the foot is left in an equinus position for a prolonged period, the Achilles tendon becomes contracted and ankle stiffness ensues.
2. At the anterior aspect of the ankle, do not allow edges of cast padding to lay immediately within the joint line.
   a. Allowing edges of cast padding to lay immediately within the joint line will create wrinkling and can lead to skin breakdown in this very fragile area.
   b. Span the area by having the mid-point of the cast padding roll directly over the ankle flexion crease; by doing so, the cast padding will be slightly tented above the joint line and will not be in direct contact with the skin, thus reducing the risk of skin breakdown.

Pearls
1. Raise the stretcher as high as it will go to make application of the cast easier.
2. Keeping the foot out of equinus sometimes can be difficult. If no reduction is necessary, placing the patient in a prone position can facilitate proper positioning of the ankle:
   a. The patient may lay prone with his or her knee bent to 90 degrees. Gravity will aid, but not completely prevent equinus.
   b. To prevent equinus with the patient prone, use the following technique:
      (1) Cut a 6-foot-long piece of 4- or 6-inch stockinette.
      (2) Put the stockinette on the patient up to the mid thigh.
      (3) Have the patient lie prone and flex his or her knee to 90 degrees.
      (4) Tie the loose end to the end of the bed, such that the ankle is out of equinus.
      (5) Apply the splint.
      (6) Once the splint is completely applied, cut the stockinette close to the ends of the splint and tuck the ends under the elastic bandage.

Equipment

1. 4-inch stockinette
2. 4-inch cast padding
3. 4- or 6-inch plaster

Basic Technique

1. Patient positioning:
   a. The patient is sitting off the end of the bed. Ensure that at least half the thigh is off the bed to allow for space between the leg and the bed.
   b. Alternatively, the patient may be placed prone with the knee flexed to 90 degrees.
2. Where to start: metatarsal heads
3. Where to finish: proximal patellar tendon
4. Where to mold: supramalleolar
5. Steps:
   a. Position the patient.
   b. Prepare a stockinette.
   c. Position the stockinette.
   d. Wrap the extremity in cast padding.
   e. Create two cuffs of cast padding (see Chapter 12).
   f. Fold down the stockinette.
   g. Prepare the plaster.
   h. Apply the plaster.
   i. Apply molding.

Detailed Technique

1. Position the patient as for a short leg cast.
   a. The patient is sitting upright and the leg is freely off the end of the bed.
   b. Make sure the patient is sitting far enough forward so there is sufficient room between the posterior calf and the end of the bed.
2. Prepare a stockinette by cutting one piece of the stockinette for the distal portion at the foot.
3. Position the stockinette.
4. Wrap the extremity in cast padding.
   a. Start as proximal as possible on the lower leg and circumferentially wrap distally to the area immediately above the lateral malleolus (Figure 14-70).
      (1) Use a standard 50% overlap technique (see Chapter 12).
      (2) Two layers of wrapping are sufficient.
   b. Span the joint line with cast padding at the anterior aspect of the ankle (see aforementioned precautions).
   c. Return to the lateral malleolus and wrap over this area.
   d. Continue distally to around the foot. Do not cover the heel at this point.
   e. Once sufficient padding has been wrapped around the malleoli and the foot, the heel can be addressed.
   f. Tear 4-inch strips of cast padding and lay them on top of the heel. Repeat several times to ensure sufficient padding.

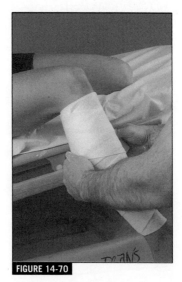

FIGURE 14-70

5. Create two cuffs of cast padding (see Chapter 12):
   a. Metatarsal heads: This cuff should form a "V" at the lateral aspect of the foot to allow for the cascade of the digits.
   b. Patellar tendon **(Figures 14-71 and 14-72):** Make sure that knee motion is unimpeded.
6. Fold down the end of the stockinette.
7. Prepare the plaster. Use the standard technique of wetting and laminating (see Chapter 12).

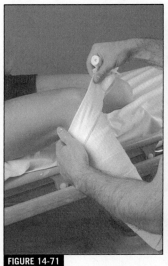

FIGURE 14-71

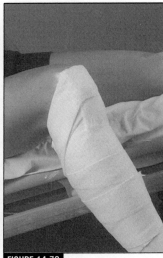

FIGURE 14-72

14

8. Apply the plaster:
   a. Start at the patellar tendon and apply a strip of 2-inch plaster over the anterior-proximal shin (Figure 14-73).
   b. Staying out of the popliteal fossa, wrap circumferential plaster to cover the strip of plaster (Figure 14-74).

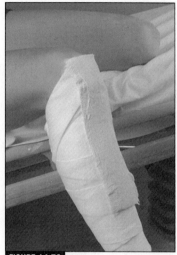

FIGURE 14-73

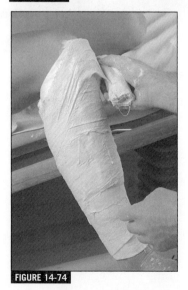

FIGURE 14-74

c. Continue wrapping as per a short leg cast. Use the standard technique of laminating while rolling (see Chapter 12).
   (1) Be vigilant about the position of the foot.
   (2) Additional thickness over the plantar aspect of the foot can be achieved by adding several precut strips, if desired.
9. Apply supramalleolar molding.
10. Make sure the cast does not limit knee flexion or extension (Figures 14-75 and 14-76).

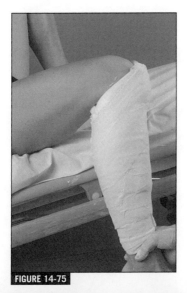

FIGURE 14-75

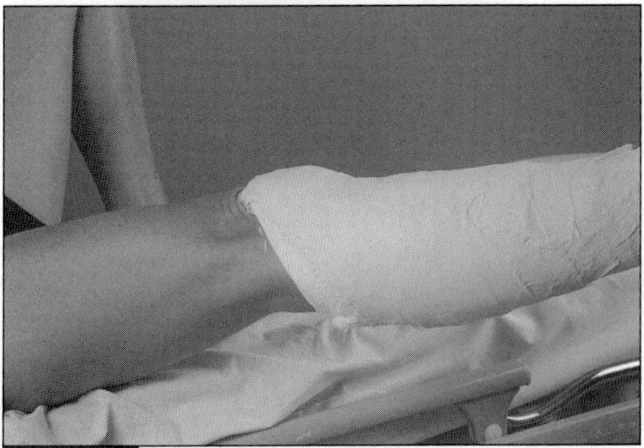

FIGURE 14-76

PART 4

TRACTION MANEUVERS

Chapter 15

Femoral Skeletal Traction

OVERVIEW

Femoral traction is accomplished with placement of a pin across the distal femur and attachment to a pulley system secured to the bed.

INDICATIONS FOR USE

1. Acetabular fractures
2. Proximal femur fractures

PRECAUTIONS

1. Do not set up femoral traction until confirming that no *skeletal* injury is present about the knee.
   a. Confirmation that no skeletal injury is present about the knee can be ascertained via a clinical examination in an alert and oriented patient or with radiographs.
   b. Note that femoral traction continues to be indicated when a *ligamentous* injury to the knee is present.
2. The pin must be inserted from the medial aspect to avoid injury to the femoral artery.
3. Ensure that the pin is placed under sterile technique. Do not place pins through or near open wounds.
4. Ensure that the pin is placed perpendicularly to the axis of the limb *and* in a straight horizontal plane.
5. Place traction weights gently!
6. Once traction has been established, ensure that the traction bow is not in contact with the skin.
   a. A pressure ulcer can be created easily by the traction bow.
   b. To ensure that the traction bow does not create a pressure ulcer, the bow should be overwrapped in rolled gauze.
7. Apply rubber stoppers or similar end caps to the ends of the pin to prevent injury to the patient or health care workers.

PEARLS

1. Close coordination with the operating surgeon is mandatory when placing patients into traction.
2. Insertion of femoral traction can be completed under local anesthetic, but conscious sedation is preferred.

3. If only a local anesthetic is being used, consider increasing the amount and adding bupivacaine.

4. If the patient is going to go to the operating room for definitive fixation shortly after placement of femoral traction, elective intubation prior to placement may be prudent.

5. Before placement of femoral traction, ensure that the patient is on a bed that is capable of having a traction frame attached to it.

6. Placement of a femoral pin is easiest when all the equipment is organized. Having two bedside tables facilitates organization and maintenance of a sterile environment.

7. Having an assistant is not mandatory but is extremely helpful.

8. A hand drill or power drill may be used. We prefer using a power drill, especially in younger patients with good bone stock.

EQUIPMENT

1. Sterile technique items:
   a. Sterile gloves
   b. 4 × 4 inch gauze
   c. Antiseptic: Chlorhexidine or Betadine
   d. Sterile drapes or blue towels
2. Local anesthesia items:
   a. Syringe: 10-mL syringe
   b. Needle:
      (1) Large-bore, blunt-tipped, drawing-up needle
      (2) 2-inch, 21-gauge needle
   c. Anesthetic: Lidocaine, 10 mL of 2%
3. Items for insertion of pin:
   a. #11 blade scalpel
   b. Straight hemostat
   c. Centrally threaded Steinmann pin (also known as a Denham nail), 4 × 225 mm or 5 × 225 mm (Figure 15-1)

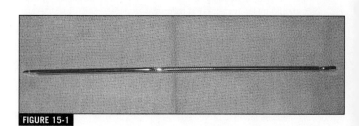

FIGURE 15-1

    d. Power drill and battery (Figure 15-2)

    e. Jacobs chuck and key (Figure 15-3)

4. Items for establishing traction:

    a. Böhler's stirrup (also known as a traction bow) (Figure 15-4)

    b. Large pin cutters

    c. Xeroform

    d. Two rubber stoppers (if specialized rubber stoppers are not available, find two blood vials and take the rubber tops off)

    e. 2 × 6 inch rolled gauze

    f. Pulley and frame: bed frame with attached single pulley

    g. Weights: six 5-lb weights with associated hanger

    h. Cord: braided traction cord

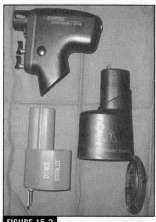

FIGURE 15-2

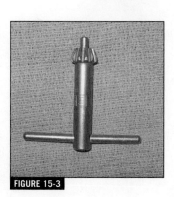

FIGURE 15-3

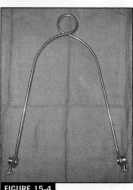

FIGURE 15-4

15

BASIC TECHNIQUE

1. Patient positioning:
   a. Ensure the patient is on a bed that accepts external frames.
   b. The patient is supine.
   c. A bump is placed under the knee.
      (1) The amount of knee flexion correlates with the desired degree of knee flexion when traction is applied.
      (2) Typically 20 degrees is sufficient.
      (3) A bump also may be placed under the thigh to prevent the leg from falling into external rotation.
2. Landmarks:
   a. Superior pole of the patella
   b. Anterior and posterior cortices of the femur
3. Steps:
   a. Ensure the patient is adequately sedated.
   b. Position the patient.
   c. Set up back tables using the sterile technique.
   d. Palpate landmarks.
   e. Prepare the skin with an antiseptic solution.
   f. Place sterile drapes.
   g. Administer local anesthesia.
   h. Insert the pin.
   i. Set up the traction apparatus.
   j. Apply traction.

DETAILED TECHNIQUE

1. Ensure the patient is adequately sedated.
2. Position the patient:
   a. Supine
   b. Place a bump under the thigh, if desired.
3. Set up back tables using the sterile technique.
   a. Open all sterile equipment, including instruments for local anesthesia.
   b. Assemble the drill (Figures 15-5 and 15-6).

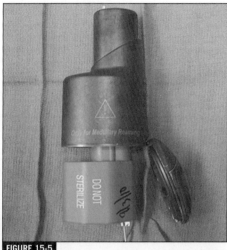

FIGURE 15-5

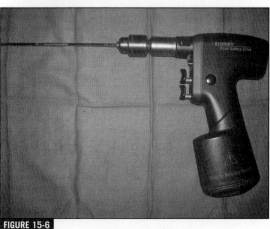

FIGURE 15-6

4. Palpate landmarks with the knee in full extension.
   a. The superior pole of the patella is palpated.
   b. The entry site is at this level, just above the mid coronal plane on the medial aspect of the limb.
   c. Mark the entry site (Figure 15-7).
5. Place a knee bump, if desired.
6. Prepare the skin with an antiseptic solution.
   a. Prepare the leg in a wide fashion.
   b. Ensure that both the medial entry site and lateral exit site are included.
      (1) It is helpful to have an assistant hold the leg in the air.
      (2) Holding the leg in the air is usually possible only if the patient is intubated.
7. Place sterile drapes.
   a. If the leg was elevated, place a sterile drape under the leg befoe draping out the relevant area.
   b. Drape out all four aspects: proximal, distal, medial, and lateral.
8. Administer local anesthesia.
   a. Prepare the anesthetic by drawing up 10 mL of 2% lidocaine.
   b. Inject the anesthetic medially and laterally.
      (1) Insert the needle 90 degrees to the skin on the medial aspect.
      (2) Advance the needle until contact is made with bone.
      (3) Aspirate the needle before injection to ensure that intravascular placement has been avoided.
      (4) Inject 2 mL directly into the bone to anesthetize the periosteum.
      (5) Withdraw the needle and continue to inject another 3 mL of anesthetic.
      (6) Repeat on the lateral aspect.

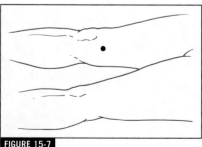

FIGURE 15-7

9. Insert the pin.
   a. Make a vertical stab incision in the skin at the entry site.
   b. Perform blunt dissection with a straight hemostat through the soft tissue to the medial cortex.
   c. Insert the Steinmann pin using the drill through the medial and lateral cortices (Figure 15-8).
      (1) The pin *must* be kept parallel to the floor to ensure it is the horizontal plane.
      (2) The pin should be inserted parallel to the knee joint line.
   d. Once the lateral soft tissue is entered with the Steinmann pin, carefully palpate where the pin will exit the skin.
   e. Make a small stab incision to allow pin passage through the lateral skin.
   f. Continue to insert the pin until equal lengths are present on either side of the limb.

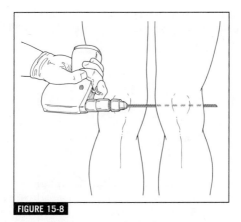

FIGURE 15-8

15

10. Set up the traction apparatus:
    a. Attach a traction bow (Figure 15-9).
    b. Cut excess length from the Steinmann pin with large pin cutters, if necessary. Hold the pin with a hemostat to prevent the cut pin fragment from becoming a flying object.
    c. Apply rubber stoppers to the ends of the pin.
    d. Wrap small strips of Xeroform around skin exit sites.
    e. Hold an unraveled roll of gauze at the apex of the bow.
    f. Wrap the entire traction bow and roll of gauze with 6-inch rolled gauze to secure the rubber stoppers and rolled gauze pad.
    g. Set up the bed frame and pulley (Figure 15-10).
    h. Attach the cord.
       (1) First, pass the cord through the pulley.
       (2) Tie the cord to the traction bow using a surgeon's knot.
       (3) Tie a slipknot in the free end (also known as an overhand knot with a draw-loop).
11. Apply traction.
    a. Hang weight from the slipknot.
    b. 20% of a patient's weight should be applied (typically 20 to 25 lb).

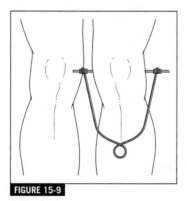

FIGURE 15-9

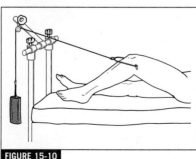

FIGURE 15-10

Chapter 16
Tibial Skeletal Traction

OVERVIEW
Tibial traction is accomplished with placement of a pin across the proximal tibial metadiaphysis and attachment to a pulley system secured to the bed.

INDICATIONS FOR USE
Femoral shaft fractures

PRECAUTIONS
1. Do not set up tibial traction until confirming that no injury is present about the knee.
   a. A clinical examination should be performed to rule out a ligamentous injury.
   b. Radiographs should be obtained prior to pin insertion.
2. The pin must be inserted from the *lateral* aspect to avoid injury to the common peroneal nerve.
3. Ensure that the pin is placed under sterile technique. Do not place pins through or near open wounds.
4. Ensure that the pin is placed perpendicularly to the axis of the limb *and* in a straight horizontal plane.
5. The Kirschner traction bow must be used with the Kirschner wire because it adds tension to the wire and prevents the wire from bending. Figure 16-1 illustrates the incorrect use of a Böhler's stirrup, resulting in a wire without tension and significantly increasing the risk of wire breakage.

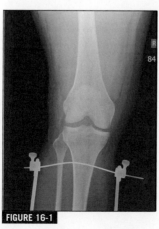

FIGURE 16-1

6. Place traction weights gently!
7. Once traction has been established, ensure that the traction bow is not in contact with skin.
   a. A pressure ulcer can be created easily by the traction bow.
   b. To ensure that the traction bow does not create a pressure ulcer, the bow should be overwrapped in rolled gauze.
8. Apply rubber stoppers to the ends of the pin to prevent injury to the patient or health care workers.

PEARLS

1. Close coordination with the operating surgeon is mandatory when placing patients into traction.
2. Insertion of tibial traction can be completed under local anesthetic, but conscious sedation is preferred.
3. If only a local anesthetic is being used, consider increasing the amount and adding bupivacaine.
4. If the patient is going to go to the operating room for definitive fixation shortly after placement of tibial traction, elective intubation prior to placement may be prudent.
5. Prior to placement of tibial traction, ensure that the patient is on a bed that is capable of having a traction frame attached to it.
6. Placement of a tibial pin is easiest when all the equipment is organized. Having two bedside tables facilitates organization and maintenance of a sterile environment.
7. Having an assistant is not mandatory but is extremely helpful.
8. A hand drill or power drill may be used. We prefer using a power drill, especially in younger patients with good bone stock.

EQUIPMENT

1. Sterile technique items:
   a. Sterile gloves
   b. 4 × 4 inch gauze
   c. Antiseptic: Chlorhexidine or Betadine
   d. Sterile drapes or blue towels
2. Local anesthesia items:
   a. Syringe: 10-mL syringe
   b. Needle:
      (1) Large-bore, blunt-tipped, drawing-up needle
      (2) 2-inch, 21-gauge needle
   c. Anesthetic: Lidocaine, 10 mL of 2%

3. Items for insertion of pin:
    a. Kirschner wire (Figure 16-2), 0.0625 inches in diameter
    b. Power drill and battery
    c. Pin driver attachment; a hand drill also may be used (Figure 16-3).
4. Items for establishing traction:
    a. Kirschner traction bow (Figure 16-4)
    b. Large pin cutters

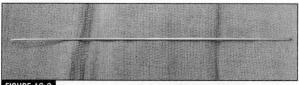

FIGURE 16-2

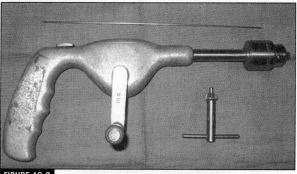

FIGURE 16-3

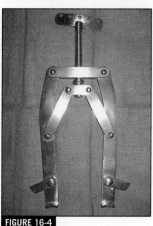

FIGURE 16-4

16

    c. Xeroform
    d. Two rubber stoppers (if specialized rubber stoppers are not available, find two blood vials and take the rubber tops off)
    e. 2 × 6 inch rolled gauze
    f. Pulley and frame: bed frame with attached single pulley
    g. Weights: six 5-lb weights with associated hanger
    h. Cord: braided traction cord

BASIC TECHNIQUE

1. Patient positioning:
    a. Ensure the patient is on a bed that accepts external frames.
    b. The patient is supine.
    c. A bump is placed under the knee.
       (1) The amount of knee flexion correlates with the desired degree of knee flexion when traction is applied.
       (2) Typically 20 degrees is sufficient.
    d. A bump also may be placed under the thigh to prevent the leg from falling into external rotation.
2. Landmarks:
    a. Tibial tubercle
    b. Anterior and posterior cortices of the tibia
3. Steps:
    a. Ensure the patient is adequately sedated.
    b. Position the patient.
    c. Set up back tables using the sterile technique.
    d. Palpate landmarks.
    e. Prepare the skin with an antiseptic solution.
    f. Place sterile drapes.
    g. Administer local anesthesia.
    h. Insert the pin.
    i. Set up the traction apparatus.
    j. Apply traction.

DETAILED TECHNIQUE

1. Ensure the patient is adequately sedated.
2. Position the patient:
    a. Supine
    b. Place a bump under the thigh, if desired.
3. Set up back tables using the sterile technique. Open all sterile equipment, including instruments for local anesthesia.

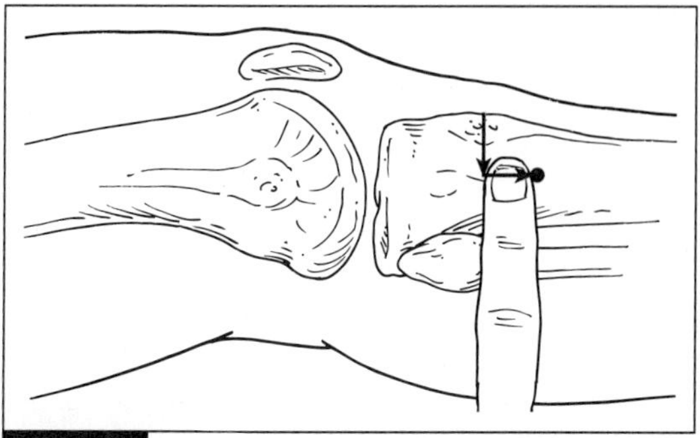

FIGURE 16-5

4. Palpate landmarks:
   a. The tibial tubercle
   b. The entry site one fingerbreadth distal and one fingerbreadth below the tibial tubercle (Figure 16-5)
5. Mark the entry site.
6. Place a knee bump, if desired.
7. Prepare the skin with an antiseptic solution.
   a. Prepare the leg in a wide fashion.
   b. Ensure that both the lateral entry site and medial exit site are included.
      (1) It is helpful to have an assistant hold the leg in the air.
      (2) Holding the leg in the air usually is possible only if the patient is intubated.
8. Place sterile drapes.
   a. If the leg was elevated, place a sterile drape under the leg prior to draping out the relevant area.
   b. Drape out all four aspects: proximal, distal, medial, and lateral.
9. Administer local anesthesia.
   a. Prepare the anesthetic by drawing up 10 mL of 2% lidocaine.
   b. Inject anesthetic laterally and medially:
      (1) Insert the needle 90 degrees to the skin on the lateral aspect.
      (2) Advance the needle until contact is made with bone.
      (3) Aspirate the needle prior to injection to ensure that intravascular placement has been avoided.
      (4) Inject 2 mL directly into the bone to anesthetize the periosteum.
      (5) Withdraw the needle and continue to inject another 3 mL of anesthetic.
      (6) Repeat on the medial aspect.

16

10. Insert the pin.
    a. Insert the Kirschner pin using the drill through the lateral and medial cortices (Figure 16-6).
       (1) The pin *must* be kept parallel to the floor to ensure that it is in the horizontal plane.
       (2) The pin should be inserted parallel to the knee joint line.
    b. Continue to insert the pin until equal lengths are present on either side of the limb.
11. Set up the traction apparatus.
    a. Attach the Kirschner traction bow (Figure 16-7).
    b. Cut excess length from the Kirschner pin with large pin cutters. Hold the pin with a hemostat to prevent the cut pin fragment from becoming a flying object.
    c. Apply rubber stoppers to the ends of the pin.
    d. Wrap small strips of Xeroform around skin exit sites.
    e. Hold unraveled rolled gauze at the apex of the bow.
    f. Wrap the entire traction bow and gauze roll with 6-inch rolled gauze to secure the rubber stoppers and rolled gauze pad.

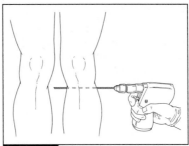

FIGURE 16-6

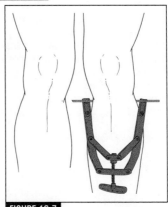

FIGURE 16-7

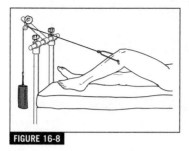

FIGURE 16-8

g. Set up the bed frame and pulley (Figure 16-8).
h. Attach the cord.
   (1) First, pass the cord through the pulley.
   (2) Tie the cord to the traction bow using a surgeon's knot.
   (3) Tie a slipknot in the free end (also known as an overhand knot
       with a draw-loop).
12. Apply traction.
    a. Hang weight from the slipknot.
    b. Twenty percent of a patient's weight should be applied (typically
       20 to 25 lb).

Chapter 17

Calcaneal Skeletal Traction

OVERVIEW

Calcaneal traction is accomplished with placement of a pin across the posterior aspect of the calcaneus and attachment to a pulley system secured to the bed.

INDICATIONS FOR USE

Tibial shaft fractures

PRECAUTIONS

1. The pin should be inserted from the *medial* aspect to avoid injury to the medial calcaneal nerve and lateral plantar nerve.
2. Ensure that the pin is placed with use of the sterile technique. Do not place pins through or near open wounds.
3. Ensure that the pin is placed perpendicularly to the axis of the limb *and* in a straight horizontal plane.
4. Place traction weights gently!
5. Once traction has been established, ensure that the traction bow is not in contact with the skin.
   a. A pressure ulcer can be created easily by the traction bow.
   b. To ensure that the traction bow does not create a pressure ulcer, the bow should be overwrapped in rolled gauze.
6. Apply rubber stoppers to the ends of the pin to prevent injury to the patient or health care workers.

PEARLS

1. Close coordination with the operating surgeon is mandatory when placing patients into traction.
2. Insertion of calcaneal traction can be completed under local anesthetic, but conscious sedation is preferred.
3. If only a local anesthetic is being used, consider increasing the amount and adding bupivacaine.
4. If the patient is going to go to the operating room for definitive fixation shortly after placement of calcaneal traction, elective intubation prior to placement may be prudent.
5. Before placement of calcaneal traction, ensure that the patient is on a bed that is capable of having a traction frame attached to it.
6. Placement of a pin is easiest when all the equipment is organized. Having two bedside tables facilitates organization and maintenance of a sterile environment.

7. Having an assistant is not mandatory but is extremely helpful.
8. A hand drill or a power drill may be used. We prefer using a power drill, especially in younger patients with good bone stock.

EQUIPMENT

1. Sterile technique items:
   a. Sterile gloves
   b. 4 × 4 inch gauze
   c. Antiseptic: Chlorhexidine or Betadine
   d. Sterile drapes or blue towels
2. Local anesthesia items:
   a. Syringe: 10-mL syringe
   b. Needle:
      (1) Large-bore, blunt-tipped, drawing-up needle
      (2) 2-inch, 21-gauge needle
   c. Anesthetic: Lidocaine, 10 mL of 2%
3. Items for insertion of pin:
   a. 15 blade scalpel
   b. Hemostat
   c. Kirschner wire, 0.0625 inches in diameter
   d. Power drill and battery
   e. Pin driver attachment
4. Items for establishing traction:
   a. Kirschner traction bow
   b. Large pin cutters
   c. Xeroform
   d. Two rubber stoppers (if specialized rubber stoppers are not available, find two blood vials and take the rubber tops off)
   e. 2 × 6 inch rolled gauze
   f. Pulley and frame: bed frame with attached single pulley
   g. Weights: six 5-lb weights with associated hanger
   h. Cord: braided traction cord

BASIC TECHNIQUE

1. Patient positioning:
   a. Ensure that the patient is on a bed that accepts external frames.
   b. The patient is supine.
   c. A bump is placed under the Achilles tendon to elevate the limb.
   d. A bump may be placed under the hip of the affected limb to internally rotate the limb.
2. Landmarks:
   a. Inferior aspect of medial malleolus
   b. Posterior-inferior aspect of calcaneus
3. Steps:
   a. Ensure that the patient is adequately sedated.
   b. Position the patient.

17

c. Set up back tables using the sterile technique.
d. Palpate the landmarks.
e. Prepare the skin with an antiseptic solution.
f. Place sterile drapes.
g. Administer local anesthesia.
h. Insert the pin.
i. Set up the traction apparatus.
j. Apply traction.

DETAILED TECHNIQUE

1. Ensure that the patient is adequately sedated.
2. Position the patient:
   a. Supine
   b. Place a bump under the hip, if desired.
3. Set up back tables using the sterile technique. Open all sterile equipment, including instruments for local anesthesia.
4. Palpate landmarks.
   a. The medial malleolus is palpated.
   b. The posterior-inferior aspect of the medial calcaneus is palpated.
   c. The entry site is posterior to the halfway point along a line from the medial malleolus to the posterior-inferior aspect of the calcaneus (Figure 17-1).
   d. Mark the entry site.
5. Prepare the skin with an antiseptic solution.
   a. Prepare the foot in a wide fashion.
   b. Ensure that both the medial entry site and the lateral exit site are included. It is helpful to have an assistant hold the leg in the air.

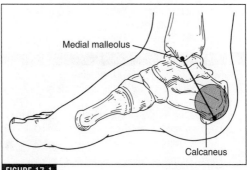

Medial malleolus

Calcaneus

FIGURE 17-1

6. Place sterile drapes.
   a. If the leg was elevated, place a sterile drape under the leg before draping out the relevant area.
   b. Drape out all four aspects: proximal, distal, medial and lateral.
7. Administer local anesthesia:
   a. Prepare the anesthetic by drawing up 10 mL of 2% lidocaine.
   b. Inject the anesthetic medially and laterally:
      (1) Insert the needle 90 degrees to the skin on the medial aspect.
      (2) Advance the needle until contact is made with bone.
      (3) Aspirate the needle prior to injection to ensure that intravascular placement has been avoided.
      (4) Inject 2 mL directly onto the bone to anesthetize the periosteum.
      (5) Withdraw the needle and continue to inject another 3 mL of anesthetic.
      (6) Repeat on the lateral aspect.
8. Insert the pin.
   a. Make a small incision in the skin at the entry site.
   b. Bluntly dissect to bone with the hemostat.
   c. Insert the Kirschner pin through the medial and lateral cortices using the drill (Figure 17-2).
      (1) The pin *must* be kept parallel to the floor to ensure that it is in the horizontal plane.
      (2) The pin should be inserted parallel to the ankle joint line.
   d. Advance the pin through the skin on the lateral aspect.
   e. Continue to insert the pin until equal lengths are present on either side of the limb.

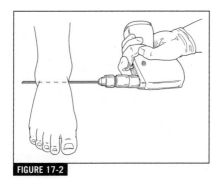

FIGURE 17-2

9. Set up the traction apparatus.
   a. Attach the traction bow.
   b. Cut excess length from the Kirschner pin with large pin cutters. Hold the pin with a hemostat to prevent the cut pin fragment from becoming a flying object.
   c. Apply rubber stoppers to the ends of the pin.
   d. Wrap small strips of Xeroform around skin exit sites.
   e. Hold an unraveled rolled gauze roll at the apex of the bow.
   f. Wrap the entire traction bow and gauze roll with 6-inch rolled gauze to secure the rubber stoppers and rolled gauze pad.
   g. Set up the bed frame and pulley.
   h. Attach the cord:
      (1) First, pass the cord through the pulley.
      (2) Tie the cord to the traction bow using a surgeon's knot.
      (3) Tie a slipknot in the free end (also known as an overhand knot with a draw-loop).
10. Apply traction.
    a. Hang weight from the slipknot.
    b. Twenty percent of a patient's weight should be applied (typically 20 to 25 lb).

Chapter 18

Cervical Spine Traction with Gardner Wells Tongs

OVERVIEW

1. Cervical spine traction is accomplished with placement of calipers or tongs to the skull and attachment to a pulley system secured to the bed.
2. Although a wide variety of tongs exist, Gardner Wells tongs are the most frequently used and the most frequently available. Gardner Wells tongs consist of a hoop attached to two 30-degree angled pins.

INDICATIONS FOR USE

1. Subaxial cervical fractures that are malaligned
2. Subaxial cervical facet dislocations
3. Selected odontoid fractures, hangman's fractures, and C1-C2 rotatory subluxation

PRECAUTIONS

1. Before application of cervical spine traction, consultation with the treating spine surgeon is paramount. Typically, unconscious or uncooperative patients require a magnetic resonance imaging (MRI) scan prior to reduction to rule out an associated disc herniation. Some controversy exists with regard to obtaining a prereduction MRI scan in patients who are awake and cooperative.
2. Repeat cervical spine radiography is essential. Use of a C-arm machine allows repeated radiography to evaluate the reduction as weights are added.
3. Careful pin placement is paramount to avoid iatrogenic injury.
4. Pin site entry is 1 cm above the pinna (earlobe) in line with the external auditory meatus.
5. Ensure that the pressure-sensitive spring-loaded indicator on the pin protrudes by 1 to 2 mm to indicate 30 inch/pounds of pressure.
6. The pins should be tightened simultaneously.
7. Traction weights need to be added cautiously and sequentially.
   a. Start with 10 lb and add 5 lb per level. For example, a C5-C6 injury should have 35 lb of traction weight.
8. Gardner Wells tongs need to be retightened after 24 hours. However, they can only be retightened once.
9. The following complications can occur with application of Gardner Wells tongs:
   a. Skull perforation
   b. Injury to the temporalis muscle or temporal artery
   c. Pin migration or pullout
   d. Infection

10. No absolute maximum weight for traction exists, but some authors suggest a limit of 70 lb. Be aware that MRI-compatible tongs are made of graphite and titanium, resulting in lower failure loads. Avoid using these tongs if more than 50 lb are to be used.

PEARLS

1. Prior to application, ensure that a complete neurologic examination is documented.
2. If an MRI scan is planned, ensure that the Gardner Wells tongs are made of MRI-compatible graphite tong and titanium pin system.
3. Place the bed into a slight reverse Trendelenburg position if the patient's weight is light and he or she slides to the top of the bed as weights are being applied.
4. Facet dislocations without associated fractures can be "unlocked" by raising the height of the pulley, thus resulting in a flexion movement and aiding in reduction.
5. Unilateral facet dislocations typically require more weight than do bilateral dislocations.

EQUIPMENT

1. A Stryker table, operative table, or other bed that is able to accept traction devices
2. Gardner Wells tongs (Figure 18-1)
3. Antiseptic: Povidone-iodine solution
4. Syringe: 10-mL syringe
5. Needle:
   a. Large-bore, blunt-tipped, drawing-up needle
   b. 1-inch, 22-gauge needle
6. Anesthetic: lidocaine, 10 mL of 2%
7. C-arm radiograph machine
8. Pulley and frame: bed frame with attached single pulley

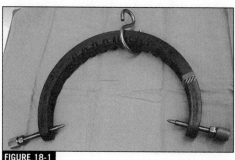

FIGURE 18-1

9. Weights:
   a. Ten 5-lb weights with associated hanger
   b. More weights may be required
10. Cord: braided traction cord

BASIC TECHNIQUE

1. Patient positioning:
   a. Place the patient supine on the table or bed.
2. Landmarks:
   a. External auditory meatus
   b. Pinna (earlobe)
   c. Insertion site: 1 cm above the pinna (earlobe) in line with the external auditory meatus
3. Steps:
   a. Position the patient.
   b. Visualize the landmarks.
   c. Prepare the skin with an antiseptic solution.
   d. Administer local anesthesia.
   e. Apply the tongs.
   f. Set up the traction apparatus (if necessary).
   g. Apply initial traction.
   h. Obtain radiographs and perform a neurologic examination.
   i. Sequentially apply traction weight until reduction is obtained and confirmed on radiographs.

DETAILED TECHNIQUE

1. Position the patient:
   a. Supine
   b. Ensure that the head of the bed can accept a traction apparatus.
2. Visualize the landmarks (Figure 18-2):
   a. Identify the pinna (top of the earlobe).
   b. Identify the external auditory meatus.
   c. Correct pin placement is 1 cm above the pinna directly in line with the external auditory meatus.

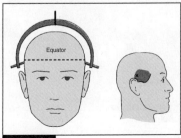

FIGURE 18-2

18

3. Prepare the skin with an antiseptic solution. Shaving is not required.
4. Administer local anesthesia:
   a. Prepare the anesthetic by drawing up 10 mL of 2% lidocaine.
   b. Inject anesthetic into each pin entry site:
      (1) Insert the needle 90 degrees to the skin.
      (2) Advance the needle until contact is made with bone.
      (3) Aspirate the needle before injection to ensure intravascular placement has been avoided.
      (4) Inject 2 mL directly into the bone to anesthetize the periosteum.
      (5) Withdraw the needle and continue to inject another 3 mL of anesthetic.
      (6) Repeat on the medial aspect.
5. Apply the tongs:
   a. Ensure that the pins are at the correct location.
   b. Simultaneously tighten the pins.
   c. One of the pins is a spring-loaded force indicator.
   d. Continue simultaneous tightening until the indicator protrudes by 1 mm (Figure 18-3).
6. Set up the traction apparatus (if necessary).
   a. Set up the bed frame and pulley if using a regular bed. The pulley should be at the same level as the patient's head.
   b. Attach the cord:
      (1) First, pass the cord through the pulley.
      (2) Tie the cord to the tongs using a surgeon's knot.
      (3) Tie a slipknot in the free end (also known as an overhand knot with a draw-loop).

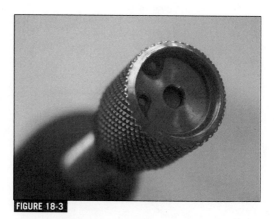

FIGURE 18-3

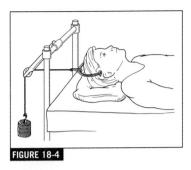

FIGURE 18-4

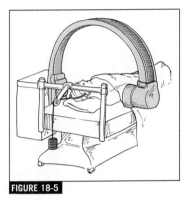

FIGURE 18-5

7. Apply initial traction (Figure 18-4). Hang 10 lb from the slipknot.
8. Obtain radiographs and perform a neurologic examination (Figure 18-5).
9. Sequentially apply traction weight until the reduction is obtained and confirmed on radiographs.
   a. Five to 10 lb are added every 20 to 30 minutes.
   b. Radiographs and a neurologic examination should be performed after each addition.

18

Index

Note: Page numbers followed by *f* indicate figures and *t* indicate tables.